Explore Your Hunger

A Guide to Hunger, Appetite, & Food

By

John Immel & Natalie Hine

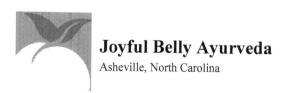

Joyful Belly Ayurveda
Asheville, North Carolina

Printed in the United States of America
First Printing, 2015

ISBN 978-1-943278-28-2

Joyful Belly Ayurveda, Inc.
PO Box 1474
Asheville, NC 28802
www.joyfulbelly.com
(828)252-0222

Contents

Acknowledgments

Introduction   9

Chapter 1: Obesity, A Modern Dilemma   17

Chapter 2: Celebrating Fat   24

Chapter 3: Your Appetite   33

Chapter 4: Taste & Food Cravings   54

Chapter 5: Experiencing Your Hunger   79

Chapter 6: The Nature of Desire   102

Chapter 7: Emotional Eating   119

Chapter 8: Food Addiction   137

Conclusion   164

Acknowledgments

We would like to thank each and every client for contributing their experiences, trials, and life stories which have been the basis for the material of this book. Ayurveda becomes possible when both the practitioner and the client are committed to sharing their stories and discovering the mysteries of our humanity. A commitment to health demonstrates love of life itself. Such great hope and faith in the heart of the client and practitioner could only be inspired by divine grace.

This book is dedicated to my children, Carmela & Elora, and to all children. May the inspirations of our generation and the love we have invested in you be the sign of hope for generations to come. We pray that the insights of this book and the mission of Joyful Belly will benefit you and your world.

We would also like to thank Joyful Belly staff for their help, contributions, and support, including David McKaig for his unabashed input & feedback.

We would like to thank our parents and the families of all Joyful Belly staff for your unwavering faith in us, even when you did not yet believe in the promise of Ayurveda. In taking such a leap of faith to support us and Ayurveda as a career choice, you create an opportunity for all people to enjoy the simple, practical gift of health.

I would like to thank John for creating Joyful Belly and freely sharing his vast knowledge on health, as well as his zeal for Ayurveda with readers around the world. You are such an inspiration to me and to many, and we are so very blessed to have your unique perspective, enthusiasm, and warmth in our lives! Thank you!

Finally I, John Immel, would like to thank you, Natalie Hine, for your extensive knowledge in the field of eating disorders, as well as your dedication, loyalty, and professionalism. Your passion for the health of our clients could only be surpassed by the joy we shared writing this book together.

Introduction

*   *   *

When you go outside and feel cold, you put on a sweater. You don't think about it, you just do it - automatically. If you get hot, you take the sweater off again. This book will teach you how to do that with food, so you won't need a list of foods or a meal plan to guide you. Instead, you can learn to trust yourself and your instincts. Just like you don't wear the same things every day, you don't eat or crave the same food every day either. One day you might naturally crave mashed potatoes and the next you may want brussel sprouts. It's a constantly changing process: you start to crave a certain ingredient, you eat it for a while, and then you stop when you've had enough. Kids do that naturally, but many adults have forgotten this skill. Thankfully, it's something you can relearn.

Clients come into our clinic every day confused about what to eat and hoping to get the perfect diet plan. But health happens naturally when you support your body; not when you force your body into a one-size-fits-all meal plan. If you have been bombarded with ads for weight loss, exercise programs, diets, and ways to recreate a better version of yourself, you will feel relieved to know that we are not presenting a new technique for you to try. True, sustainable health and weight loss won't come from a new technique or a new diet - it has to come from within. If you have been baffled by a dizzying array of "nutrition" advice, you will discover through Ayurveda your capacity to have an easy, intuitive relationship with food without relying on experts. Many weight loss scams promise a quick fix at the expense of your health. Ayurveda takes a slower approach, balancing weight goals with the integrity of your system as a whole. Ayurveda challenges you to believe that your healthiest weight is a natural byproduct of listening to your body and honoring your true hungers.

To fully benefit from the methods introduced here, there are certain beliefs and principles that will facilitate your success. You must first and foremost believe in your body. Believing in your body means you believe your body is your friend and ally, not your enemy. It means you believe that your body, not your mind, is the best tool for helping you lose weight and regain your health. You must be willing to give up the mentality of fighting with your body, and start listening to it instead. This may seem counter-intuitive if your body is telling you to eat chips, candy, or cheesecake. But by the end of this book, you will come to know that the opposite is true. You will discover that these cravings provide valuable information about your body and state of balance. You will discover that the path to weight loss is working with your food cravings and becoming aware of your body. Even if weight loss is not your goal, you will find that listening to and becoming aware of your body can benefit your health in innumerable ways.

You could take a pill to lose weight, get lap band surgery, or start a crash diet. But these techniques won't help you grow beyond the behaviors and thought patterns that created the illness in the first place. Though perhaps hard to believe, weight gain is usually a symptom, not a cause of your troubles. To lose weight you must always treat the cause, not the outcome. You may believe you need extraordinary mental discipline to battle your appetite, but unless you treat the real causes of your unruly cravings, these causes will continually undermine your willpower. If low metabolism is making you gain weight, treat your metabolism not your waistline. If emotions are behind your tendency to overeat, address your emotions instead of your food cravings. To lose weight and keep it off, you must look beyond the simple goal of shedding extra pounds and start addressing the root causes.

The word Ayurveda translates to the art and study of life, making Ayurveda unique among world systems of medicine because its scope reaches beyond fighting disease to discovering how to care for your body so that you will have a happy, healthy life. This scope includes cultivating the right perspectives, behaviors and lifestyle that will help make self-care easier for you. The result is a healing as opposed to a simple cure. A cure can help you shed a few pounds. In a true healing, you lose weight, but also grow personally and come to a new understanding about how to live well so that you never gain the weight back again. A healing is greater than a cure because it brings new wisdom and perspective, and addresses the root cause. A healing puts an end to the cycle of yo-yo diets, and the constant up and down of your weight. A successful application of Ayurveda yields this type of deeper healing from within, instead of mere weight loss.

Your healing journey starts with listening to your body. Normally, people trying to lose weight struggle to resist their food cravings, and to avoid certain foods like carbs or fats. This struggle amounts to a "fight" with your body. But you cannot heal when you wage a war against yourself. Instead of fighting your cravings, try learning from them. Instead of focusing on willpower, start by building awareness of your cravings. This is what it means to listen to your body. By examining your cravings, you will start to understand them in a whole new light. Then you will discover you were craving the chips, candy, and cheesecake for a reason. You will discover the real craving behind the 'false' one for chips. When you find this hidden reason, you will also learn what your body (and your mind) truly needs to feel satisfied. This is how following your unruly & pesky food cravings can lead you down the path to a healing.

True health starts with building a loving relationship with your body. Many people believe that loving their body means convincing themselves they are beautiful enough, athletic enough, or smart enough. They make a list of their positive attributes and try to focus on that, while ignoring their 'bad' parts. We'd like to challenge this idea of love. It's easy to love your good parts. Anybody can make a list of the things they love about themselves. But what about loving the parts of your body that you feel ashamed about? How do you do that? A person focused on being thin might ask, "How could I possibly love my fat?"

In a biblical sense, to love something means to adopt it. To love your body means to adopt it. You don't even have to like your body to love it, or your fat either. To adopt your body means to choose your body over any other, and to select it as your own. It also means to invest your time, love, and attention into caring for it, just as you would if you were adopting a child. Even if your child has many flaws or has a personality that clashes with your own, you would never exchange it for another. When you adopt a child, it becomes your own no matter what. To adopt your body means to believe in it and to place your hope in it. In adopting your body, you also come to believe that God loves your body.

Adopting your flaws and shortcomings is more difficult than it sounds. Some people look in the mirror and the person they see doesn't match their expectation. I had a client who would say, "My body is being ridiculous right now" and "my body looks like this because of the antidepressants I'm taking." When she spoke, it was as if her body was a separate entity, and unworthy of her. Inside, she knew that she was more beautiful than her reflection in the mirror. Each and every one of us has a certain beauty within, a place inside where we believe we are made in the image of God, and that place is the soul. First you feel the beauty of the soul inside of you, and then you notice that your body isn't a good representative of this inner beauty. That makes you want to reject your body, and lose hope that you can ever change. Eventually you realize the body can't, and never will, measure up to your beauty within. Initially, this realization feels like a crushing blow and you want to escape somehow. Later, you realize that nobody and nothing on earth could possibly measure up to your beauty within. There is nothing good enough to represent the inner beauty of your soul - no job, no spouse, no home, no fancy car, and no body size will measure up. You realize that to live well on earth you need to forgive your body for its shortcomings. Compassion for these shortcomings wells up from your heart as you learn to adopt many things as your own, not just your body. Adopting your loved ones, your community, your society, and nation despite their flaws and shortcomings makes your life special, tender, and sweet. You come to realize that despite their earthly shortcomings, each of these individuals has a beautiful soul too.

That is the way you must approach your body - with a spirit of adoption. Fighting your weight amounts to self-criticism. It is the opposite of adoption, which is alienation. Fighting yourself is an odd way to heal. Instead, try getting to know, understand, and appreciate how your body came to be what it is. The best way to approach your body is with awe and wonder. When you love your body, you become curious about it. Your curiosity leads you to a lighthearted adventure of self-discovery, as opposed to an endless battle against the enemy. When you love and adopt your body, you can begin to discover the curious mysteries it holds. In Ayurveda, if you wish to heal the disease as opposed to just 'curing' it, you have to start with appreciating the complexity of your imbalances rather than fighting them.

But, the journey to health takes time. In healing, the tortoise will always outrun the hare. Your body will find the weight that it should be without too much effort on your part, except the effort to know yourself. Developing body awareness is a journey over many years. Through each personal discovery you make about your body, you will notice your energy & vitality naturally increasing. Feelings and sensations that were once mysterious suddenly become clear - you start to understand them, how they are related, and how to respond to them wisely.

How will you achieve this newfound body awareness? Through your senses. Ayurveda originates from ancient India, in a time before modern technology and modern machines. All people had were their five senses to use as a guide. Like the ancient Ayurvedic sages, you can use your five sense organs to learn about your body. This book will outline how to use your senses to understand your relationship to food. The keystone to a good relationship with food is an exploration of how your body experiences food, both the eating of food and its effects on your body afterwards. Chili peppers make you sweat. Lemonade is refreshing. A hearty roast warms you up on a cold day. In Ayurveda, the different experiences you have with each food are the actual medicinal effects used to create your healing.

In addition to your experiences of food, you will also explore the many varieties, nuances, and origins of hunger. Instead of battling your food cravings, you will delve into them with curiosity, wonder, and a sense of adventure. Through this process of self-examination you will learn how emotions, your body, and hunger are inextricably linked, and how you can manage some of the deep forces within that drive your decisions and behavior around food.

Ayurveda is not a body of knowledge you can find in a library. It's an experience. It's the art of paying attention to your experiences, interpreting them and responding appropriately. It is much more than following a list of specific foods, which is a common way people approach Ayurveda. Food lists may offer helpful suggestions, but if you follow them blindly, you will stop listening to your body and the food lists will become an obstacle to your progress. So do not get hung up on technicalities, food lists, and dietary regimens, but focus on your hunger, food cravings, and getting honest about your relationship with food. The most important thing is your authenticity - knowing your body so well that you know what to eat, because you have examined your hunger and food cravings.

Many people who struggle with their weight eat food without paying much attention to it and barely even tasting it. Before you can lose weight, you have to begin truly tasting food, as though for the first time. You have to appreciate food as though it were cuisine rather than mere provision, savoring the taste of food and experiencing its effects on your body directly. Many people believe that enjoying food is incompatible with weight loss, but our experience suggests the opposite. People gain weight because they don't enjoy food enough or take the time to savor it. They simply consume it. Through Ayurveda you become a kind of connoisseur of food, able to appreciate the subtle effects of it on your body and able to use food to take care of yourself.

My own journey to awareness and health was slow. I came to Ayurveda with severe digestive problems resulting from years of travel overseas. It took me years to fully appreciate exactly how Ayurveda could help me. It happened in many small eureka moments where I would suddenly realize something about myself or my health. It is important to stay focused on those rather than your weight. When you focus on moments of discovery and your small successes each day, you will be learning about yourself, and little by little your body will shift and you will become a healthier, more vibrant version of yourself. And, the process will be much more fun than dieting, counting calories, or restricting yourself to a food list.

Chapter 1: Obesity, A Modern Dilemma

*

   Obesity has become a leading "preventable" cause of death worldwide but was rare before the twentieth century. Preventable is in quotes because we recognize that if obesity was simple to prevent, we wouldn't need to write this book. In reality, we all know what a struggle it is to lose weight, especially given our modern lifestyle, food, and culture. Some individuals struggle to lose weight for years and years with variable success. For many, this battle elicits feelings of frustration or hopelessness. They conclude that their body has a flaw in its design or construction - that they were born "big boned" and doomed forever. Rest assured, the difficulty they are experiencing as they try to lose weight is not simply a personal failure.

   In light of what is happening globally, you will be pleased to know your body isn't the problem; it's the changes around you. The issue of disordered weight gain is a new phenomenon and widespread. Thousands of years ago, the capacity to gain weight was a selective advantage, evolutionarily-speaking. It was a life-saving skill to help your ancestors survive famines, which were all too frequent. In modern times, however, the resourceful tendency to gain weight has become more problematic. In 1977, the World Health Organization

(WHO) formally recognized obesity as a global epidemic. By 2008, the WHO reported that five million adults, over 10% of the population, are obese in both developing and industrialized nations.

What has changed? What is it about modern lifestyle that makes weight gain a problem rather than a lifesaving advantage? Perhaps it is because we have become more sedentary. We are less likely to be out working in the fields and more likely to be sitting at a desk, behind a computer, or on a sofa. This means we burn less calories but still have the same appetite and food cravings as our ancestors did. We also put much less energy into acquiring and preparing our food. Historically, finding food was much less convenient and required a lot of work. It wasn't pre-packaged on a shelf for easy consumption like it is today. Our ancestors exerted significant physical effort just to eat even a simple meal: growing, hunting, gathering, canning, naturally preserving, and even cooking took up a large portion of life in the past. There was no drive-thru where you could pick up a quick meal if you didn't feel like cooking one night. There was no canned soup, packaged dinners, or frozen pizza either - everything had to be harvested and prepared, by hand and from scratch.

Not to mention that we have distanced ourselves from the farms and fields where food is grown. Unlike our ancestors, we are more likely to purchase our food and produce from the local supermarket than from the farmer down the road. It makes sense that our connection with food seems more abstract. As an herbalist I am always struck by how much easier it is to understand an herb after encountering it in the wild, and seeing the whole plant rather than the powdered extract.

It is similarly difficult to understand the effects of food without knowing the living plant or animal it came from, as well as its growing conditions.

According to *Mindful Eating,* the only place where obesity is rare is sub-Saharan Africa, where people still live in hunter-gatherer tribes. They have to work hard for their meals, chasing wild game and foraging for berries and vegetables. Their food is nutritionally dense and high in fiber, plus it is devoid of empty carbohydrates, artificial sweeteners, preservatives, and some of the other processed foods that plague modern civilization. Food in these regions is pure, simple, and unprocessed, and requires significant physical exertion from the people to harvest and prepare.

A major reason for the obesity epidemic is modern food processing, too much refined flours, and the availability of refined sugars, all of which has had an enormous impact on our health and weight. Advanced preservation techniques have made richer, sweeter foods more accessible at any time. Before modern refrigeration, you couldn't have ice cream whenever you wanted it. Before preservatives, sugary food would quickly rot and turn rancid. But today, preservatives allow for a constant supply of processed sugar-rich foods. For many Americans, sugary drinks or sodas constitute 25% of daily calories.

In modern times, we consume about 150 times the amount of sugar that our ancestors did. King Henry of England once boasted a royal feast featuring three pounds of sugar as the sign of opulent luxury, a quantity he struggled to obtain.[1] Now you can easily acquire 10

---

1 Leonard Alfred George Strong, *The Story of Sugar* (London: Weidenfeld & Nicolson, 1954), 67.

pounds of sugar for about $5.50. The profound contrast between the ancestral rarity of sweet taste, and the modern abundance of it, is an affront to your biological design, much like the thawing of the last Ice Age must have felt to a woolly mammoth who no longer needed a thick coat of fur.

The American Heart Association states that your body can handle about 6 teaspoons of sugar a day, or 24 grams. This is half the amount of sugar in one can of Coca Cola. We believe that this is still just way too much sugar for one person. While each body is different, Ayurveda claims that your body is designed to handle only about 2 teaspoons of added sugar per day. This includes raw sugar, table sugar, honey, fructose, and agave nectar. The artificial alternatives like Splenda and Sweet-N-Low are not calorie-free choices you can eat in abundance - in fact, they might just be worse for you.[2]

There is another major reason for modern weight gain. The last 100 years has seen a dramatic increase in the use of pharmaceutical or prescription drugs. Many of these pharmaceuticals lead to weight gain because they cause water retention, slow down digestion, or trigger depression. Many women are also having children later in life, and pregnancies in later life are statistically shown to produce higher weight children. It seems that modern life, given all these factors, makes gaining weight and having a larger body size much easier and perhaps even more normal.

There are environmental factors that contribute to weight gain as well, such as air conditioning. Air conditioning thwarts natural changes in your appetite

---

2 Holly Strawbridge. "Artificial sweeteners: sugar-free, but at what cost?," *Harvard Health Blog,* July 2012.

that help you adapt to the seasons. Climate control is especially problematic if you are trying to lose weight in summer months. As the weather heats up in the summer, your body adjusts to keep cool. Your appetite naturally wanes as the temperature increases. Internal biological mechanisms cause you to purge a layer of insulating winter fat from your body once the weather gets hot. But if you sit in air conditioning all day, your body won't adjust to the season. It won't let go of winter weight, your winter eating habits won't change, and you won't lose those extra seasonal pounds as easily.

In July, when the temperature begins to peak at 100 degrees, most people run to crank up the AC. In January, when the temperature drops below freezing, most people turn up the furnace. These peak extremes are ideal times to go for a walk outside and experience the seasonal variety of nature. Nature's yearly drama is the temperature changes through all four seasons. Fully experiencing that will keep you healthy. Experiencing the high peaks and low valleys of temperature and humidity keeps you refreshingly connected with your environment. Take precaution when you spend time in these extremes if you have a medical condition.

Unless you are obese, you are also programmed to gain weight in the winter. Most people gain 8 - 11 pounds in the winter, depending on where they live, and lose it again in the spring and summer months - that's normal and natural. I have seen many clients who are scared of gaining weight in the fall, and eat a diet that is so lean it compromises the strength of their immune system. They catch a nasty cold in November that seems to last all winter long. It's not healthy to try to resist your body's seasonal rhythms. Rest assured, you will shed those pounds again once spring rolls around if you listen to your body.

In addition to adjusting the amount of insulating fats with the seasons, you'll start to notice how your body directs you towards healthy food habits for each season of the year. For example, your craving for hot chocolate and sitting by the fireside comes right on time in December. Such an act would be unthinkable in June, when you are more likely to crave cooling foods like watermelon or freshly-squeezed lemonade. In October, you might perk up at the sound of warm apple cider or sautéed butternut squash, while March cravings may look more like salads, asparagus & fresh herbs like parsley. These cravings are actually supportive and can keep you balanced and healthy through the seasons.

Your body is programmed to crave certain foods with each season. If you are ever unsure or confused about what to eat to stay healthy, go outside. If you spend too much time indoors, you will be confused about what to eat. The great outdoors will sharpen your body's awareness of how to eat healthy with the seasons. You'll need just enough time outdoors to adjust to the temperature. My own body adjusts to the climate after about a half hour or so outside. Everybody is different, so it may take yours fifteen minutes or three hours to make the same adjustment. You'll know your body is adjusted to the temperature when you feel comfortable. You've probably had the experience of stepping outside in the winter and feeling uncomfortably blasted by the cold. But after a half hour of walking you feel fine & adjusted. At the point where you feel comfortable, your body is fully aware of the season. Of course, you must be dressed properly for this experiment as well.

After your outdoor experience, you'll notice your cravings are sharper - you will know intuitively what to eat. To stay in tune with the season, you'll need at least an hour outdoors each week. For an Ayurvedic practitioner, spending more time outside can help you truly absorb the wisdom of nature and the seasons. You will be more helpful and insightful as you guide your clients towards what to eat during that time of the year, just by spending a little bit of time outdoors.

With simple techniques like this one to tune your body into seasonal changes and reconnect to nature, surviving modern changes will suddenly seem easier. Ayurveda can show you many more tools to tune your instincts, all of which will help you collaborate with your body and return to a state of balanced equilibrium and weight. Along the way you'll develop a heightened awareness of your body, so that your relationship with food will seem less mysterious.

Chapter 2: Celebrating Fat

*

Throughout history, weight has often been a sign of health and prosperity. To be a little on the heavier side was considered to be a good thing; having a few extra pounds was prized and considered attractive. A hearty woman would make it through cold winters, difficult childbirths, and would have a long life. Burly men were seen as strong and able, protecting their families and forging a fruitful livelihood in the fields. Fat was a sign of wealth, prosperity, and also fertility. Ayurveda agrees that a bit of extra weight can be healthy and desirable. Ayurveda considers fat luxurious, sweet, and loving.

In India, the Sanskrit word for love and the word for oil are the same: *sneha*. "Fat" literally means love in India. In English, we have proverbs like "buttering someone up" and "greasing the wheels," both indicative of oil's power to make a person feel happy and loved. Ayurveda believes fat is necessary for stable-bonded love. This is because fat is affectionate; it is loving and heart-warming. Fat calms a person, and makes them feel stable. A little bit of fat in your diet satisfies your appetite so you don't feel hungry all the time. Fat is comfortable and secure. It is the stable layer of protection that gets you through the cold winter, or life's ups and downs. The last thing you want to do is fight it. You simply want to balance it, if it has become excessive.

You shouldn't fight to lose a few pounds. It's a pop-culture phenomenon to feel extremely anxious about being overweight, an impulse you should certainly resist. If you have an inch to pinch, that's OK. Not only is it ok, but it is actually beneficial! I have a friend who was lucky to have a healthy body weight and an inch to pinch. She went abroad to Mexico, got a parasite, and lost 20 pounds very quickly. She lost so much weight, she almost died. If she didn't have the 20 pound to lose in the first place, she might never have survived. Fat saved her. Without that buffer, the world is a scary, dangerous place.

This woman had a male friend who saw her after the parasite episode at her absolute thinnest. He told her, "Wow, you look reeeeeeaally good." She reports, "I about socked him in the face and laid in about how I almost died and how women are supposed to have fat." Comments like these from others might seem to justify excessive compulsion to lose weight. You might feel, "I have to lose weight to succeed. If I were skinny, men would notice me more." But, it's important to take these comments with a grain of salt. There are many reasons to compliment a person for losing weight, beyond mere beauty or attractiveness. Losing weight is hard work. Her male friend might have been simply acknowledging what he believed was her hard work, not her attractiveness. Heartier woman might not get compliments for gaining weight simply because it is not as socially unacceptable to compliment a woman for gaining weight or being voluptuous, even when men find them attractive.

Since the 1920's, the culturally ideal weight has dropped dramatically and models have gotten skinnier and skinnier. At the same time, there has been a steep increase in average body weight. It seems that the heavier we have become as a nation, the more we have idealized thinness. As food becomes more conveniently available, it becomes harder to resist. In response, controlling appetite has become a new cultural ideal as well.

Naturally, if you have too much fat, it poses a health problem. Obesity causes a strain on your heart and your body, making weight loss important for an obese person's overall health. Whether or not you actually need to lose weight, Ayurveda suggests a gentle approach. Don't obsess over it. Choose to be healthy. Choose to examine your food cravings. When you are eating healthfully and taking good care of yourself, your body will figure out what weight is healthy for you and self-regulate. Your body works well when you work with it, not against it.

So how much fat is healthy? Ayurvedically speaking, all of the "ideal weight" statistics are misleading because they assume the ideal is the same for every body type. In Ayurveda, the optimum weight for a person really depends on the individual and the individual's constitution. You have a unique constitution - a unique composition, structure, and configuration of genetic and environmental factors that have shaped and formed you. Your unique construction behaves and responds differently to food and weight than others. Some people (typically those with a Vata type in Ayurveda) are overweight at the medically recommended average. Others may be underweight (typically Kapha) at this average. Figure out what feels good for your constitution. And if it feels good, own it and adopt it. That's what's going to be supportive to your body and well-being.

There are problems with following these cultural ideals of thinness and self-control. Controlling your appetite means not listening to your body. Instead of brute force control, examine your appetite and reconnect to it, so you won't mindlessly reach for a donut or empty carbs. Rather than look to confusing societal norms to define your weight loss goals, ask yourself, "what weight makes me feel healthy, stable, and vital? What weight feels good on me and my unique body?" Your answer should not be a number or a look that will silence those critical voices in your head. Instead, determine what weight feels good physically, not what you believe makes you "look good." When you are your healthiest weight, others will naturally be attracted to your glow of health.

As you ask these questions, you might discover you are reading this book because you have a vision of your ideal weight which is completely disconnected from your actual welfare and happiness, and that you don't need to lose weight at all. If that's the case, Ayurveda can help you too - by guiding you through the process of reconnecting to hunger and healthy food cravings. A client relates her process of discovering her ideal weight:

> *I lost too much weight and didn't understand why. I was working too hard, eating too little. I also had a chronic illness. When I told my doctor that I had dropped all these pounds so fast, he said, "That's a normal side effect of your illness, to gain and lose weight due to depression." Outside of the doctor, I was constantly complimented on my weight. Even one nurse asked me while I was being weighed*

at a doctor's appointment, "How do you stay so thin?" I was 5'2" and 90 pounds. Obviously anyone, especially in the medical world should have expressed concern, not dished out compliments.

Eventually, I was diagnosed with a parasite and treated. I immediately started gaining weight and was so relieved to have found a solution to the weight loss. There was a surprise though - I didn't realize how deeply connected my anxiety and depression was to my weight loss. I thought these emotions were related to my overall ailing health, not to being underweight. As I began to gain weight, I slowly started to notice that I wasn't as anxious or emotionally unstable. I stopped taking medication for anxiety and depression. Now I feel happy and stable. This is the weight that feels good to me.

It might take some time to retrain your mental outlook before you can sense what weight feels good on your body. The media influences women to feel that they are not beautiful or attractive unless they are unattainably thin. This image is impossible to achieve without restriction. It leaves women feeling extremely insecure, ugly, and fat even at a healthy weight. It makes them feel like they must overcome their natural appetite for food; that there is something wrong with their bodies, with their hunger.

Excessive preoccupation with the body, its weight or health, often has its roots in fear of being alone, undesirable, or unsuccessful. Modern culture tempts you to think that a sexy or otherwise attractive body is your ticket to love and happiness. Seeing rail-thin models on the cover of magazines or on television commercials, smiling and laughing, creates an illusory association between happiness and skinniness. But, at the end of the day, it is an act of faith to believe that your heart is the main source of attraction, rather than your body. Cultivating a belief that your heart is what makes you valuable, even if you don't believe it at first, is crucial to releasing the preoccupation with body size and weight.

If you believe thin people are happier, take note of this statistic. A study of 1,979 overweight adults by the University College of London reports that individuals who lost more than 5% of their body weight were 78% more likely to suffer from depression. In another study of 169 married couples by Southern Methodist University, they report that happily married couples are typically heavier than their unhappy counterparts. This research implies that an extra inch to pinch may be a happier choice. Note that despite these statistics, obesity (a much more extreme condition than being overweight) also increases depression. There is a clear connection between mood and weight.

As you start to appreciate the love and happiness that a few extra pounds of weight have brought to your life, you might discover that your relationship with food is a part of your personality and how you live your life. For example, some of my clients are overweight because they enjoy making people happy by cooking for them. They want to create an atmosphere of hospitality and affection with food. They love to bake cakes and cookies for the people in their lives. Asking them to eat a lean weight loss friendly diet would mean disappointing their loved ones. Other clients of mine try so hard not to disappoint their co-workers that they work long hours without a break, leaving little time and attention for personal health. These issues aren't physical in nature, but are wholly psychological. Your eating patterns are closely connected to your priorities, values, and belief systems, whether you are aware of them or not.

When life feels harsh, like a string of traumatic events in a row that are just too hard to manage, you may crave sweets not because you are hungry but because sweet foods can soothe and abate some of the painful emotions you are experiencing. Maybe you are working through difficult issues with children or your spouse. On some days, eating a cookie seems to help you cope with life's inevitable ups and downs, and provides temporary relief from stress. Those cookies do add much needed sweetness to the moment, and seem to give you a little more patience. There is no fault in craving sweetness, and no fault in seeking comfort, even in the occasional cookie. However, using food to soothe your emotions can lead to weight and health imbalances, and ultimately does not bring the true emotional sweetness that you crave.

Cravings are the emotions of your body. When you crave a particular taste, it corresponds to an emotion you are having. By eating the food, you are not only satisfying your body, but you are also providing emotional relief as well. Reaching for something sweet when you feel crazed or out of control can ground you. Through food, you can "sweeten" the moment or bite away the anger. In other words, your sugar cravings might be due as much to your emotions as they are to your tongue. Tastes aren't simply biological. The body and mind are connected.

Being overweight is sometimes the shadow side of an affectionate personality. Many of us have a tendency to binge a bit on sweets when we feel the need to be sweet. Your belief in treating others sweetly on a psychological level, especially if it is a denial or suppression of your true tendencies, can create a biological craving to eat sweet things. It could even be that you overvalue a personality of sweetness. We all love a kind, generous grandmother. Or the sweet neighbor who carefully and affectionately takes their dog out for a walk each day, rain or shine. You might feel inspired to imitate these lovely qualities yourself, and express your nurturing side more generously. You may have noticed that sweetness comes naturally to you. Maybe you identify with being a loving, heart-warming person. Sweetness may be your gift. If that translates into the food you eat, meaning that you tend to reach for sweet things that mirror your sweet and loving personality, it can create a love/hate relationship with sweets that seems all too difficult to resist.

What if you've based your whole personality on being sweet? If you gave up sugar then who would you be? Suddenly, giving up sugar seems risky. You might fear losing the affection of loved ones. You might feel like you are giving up your whole identity if you give up sweets, and that sugar is your soul food. It's not just about the sweet taste itself, but also about the belief that runs much deeper than that - it's at the core of your identity.

Maybe you provide stability, nurture, and protection for others and you eat comfort food whenever that security is threatened. Whenever one feels a little insecure, fat and sugar provides reassurance. In those instances, giving up sweets could mean giving up who you are. It's not just a food addiction; it's a belief system and a lifestyle. It's bigger than a food addiction. Your investment in sweetness can be a blessing and a curse because you recognize the positive response you get from others. But the negative consequence is gaining weight. You might need a solution that doesn't throw out the baby with the bathwater. Through this book, you will discover a way of maintaining your sweetness without affecting your waistline.

Chapter 3: Your Appetite

*

Appetite is the desire to eat food. The size of your appetite determines how much you eat. If you eat when you lack appetite, it leads to overeating and often weight gain. Young children naturally do not overeat. Many are the toddler who picks at his food for days on end, leaving the nervous parents wondering why he won't eat and how he could develop and grow on so little food. This is because children under the age of five are often still in tune with their appetite. Children allow their appetite to tell them when to start and stop eating.

A child under five does not have preconceived food preferences, memories of past food experiences, or learned habits overriding their natural intuition about food. Not too long ago, when my daughter was two years' old, she would often ask for a banana, repeating her request over and over again. Finally relenting, I would peel her banana. After a single, thoughtful bite, she would hand it back saying, "Daddy, I don't want a banana." She had imagined she wanted a banana, but her taste of the banana contradicted her imagination. Of course, the peeled banana was of no use to anyone at that point. Yet, the innocence of her cravings was refreshingly impulsive - she was truly in the moment with her food.

After about 5 years old, children start to anticipate the food they want from memory. The mind is greedy to replicate the past joy of eating a cupcake or candy. As you grow up, these memories continue to override your internal gut impulses until as an adult you may be eating based on memories, instead of what you truly need to nourish yourself. Eating this way, disconnected from your actual experience, will leave you thoroughly mystified about what foods to eat. Fortunately, even if you are in the habit of ignoring hunger and satiation cues, you have the capacity to reconnect to your true appetite and improve your awareness of it, so you can eat like a 5 year old. Once you know your true appetite, you'll know exactly how much and which foods your body truly needs.

Sometimes, regulating your appetite becomes confused with the catchphrase "portion control." The implication hidden in 'portion control' is that exerting willful control over your body will help you stop overeating. By willfully controlling portions (or at least attempting to), you are using your mind to overcome the will of the body instead of learning to listen to your body. That is the mind telling the body, "I control you." Instead, trust your body. Through body awareness you can safely regulate your appetite. Your body has the capacity to decide the proper portion for you, but sometimes due to habit or poor food choices, your appetite becomes distorted. Rather than criticizing your appetite, consider some of the ways in which you might have harmed your appetite or ignored your own limits. Reflect on your hunger and desire to eat. Ultimately it is body awareness, not willful control, which will lead to a stable long term solution to overeating.

Understanding the biology behind your appetite can help you develop appetite intuition & awareness. The intensity of your appetite is due to four internal mechanisms. One mechanism is the physical sensation of emptiness and fullness. When your stomach is empty, it grumbles and you feel hungry. As it starts to fill up, nerves that monitor pressure in your stomach wall send a signal to your brain that makes you feel full. Second, your appetite is affected by the amount of nutrients in your bloodstream. If you don't have enough glucose, fats, amino acids, vitamins, and minerals, you will feel hungry. If you have enough of these nutrients you will feel satisfied. There are also several hunger-abating hormones that tell your body when you are full, such as cholecystokinin, insulin, and glucagon. These hormones are released by the small intestine and pancreas. Finally, the fat cells themselves release leptin and other chemicals to turn off your hunger.

It's important to notice all the different sensations of hunger and fullness in your gut. You can feel the difference between the four bio-mechanisms above. When your stomach is full but your blood sugar level is low, you feel pressure without satisfaction. When your blood is well nourished on the other hand, you feel satisfied. The release of hormones in your small intestine makes the thought of more food slightly nauseating. Finally, when your fat cells release leptin, food seems to lose its appeal altogether. Pay attention to each of these nuances of feeling full, and you will be less likely to overeat.

With so many hormones and feedback mechanisms to help you feel your appetite, it should seem easy and instinctive to regulate portion. Unfortunately, it's not that simple. Your appetite may be distorted by pharmaceuticals. Or, pain in the stomach can make you feel hungry when you aren't. More frequently, your appetite becomes habituated to incorrect eating habits. Many people simply don't pay attention. They forget to notice, and at times even suppress, the full feeling in their belly.

Some people feel a certain pride in stuffing another bite down the hatch despite the cries of their stomach. They feel a macho sense of accomplishment, a kind of "I can do it!" I was watching the Barbara Streisand movie *Guilt Trip* a few weeks ago. Halfway through the movie, they stop for dinner at a Texan BBQ and win the giant steak eating contest. Have you ever seen a contest like that? There are many variations, such as "Win a FREE T-SHIRT if you can eat this monster burrito," or "If you can eat this gallon-sized banana split sundae, it's FREE." Restaurant owners know the sense of pride and accomplishment you feel ignoring your body and conquering a large meal.

Perhaps this is true mostly for men, but as a boy I used to boast about my appetite. I could drink an entire Big Gulp from 7-11. I could eat a whole pizza pie. My mom would cook a pound of pasta for the family, and a pound for me. Macho portions made me feel big and powerful, like others must feel after a "Hungry Man Breakfast." Somehow, the feeling that I could dominate a meal appealed to me as a budding man. Whenever I ate that whole pound of pasta or pizza pie, I never considered what happened to the food after I ate it or how much it must have distended my stomach (a scary thought to me now!). Before I studied Ayurveda, I ate as much as I possibly could every meal because I enjoyed the satisfaction of fullness. Several months into studying Ayurveda, I realized my stomach actually wasn't working that well when stuffed. I was having trouble digesting my food. Once I started paying attention to fullness, I ate less. My digestion improved and consequently, my overall health improved. It was a revelation.

Ayurveda suggests that you heed your body's appetite when it tells you that you are "at capacity." Take the time to notice when you're not enjoying the taste of the food anymore, which is a sure sign that it's time to stop eating. Eating beyond your body's appetite limitations is an inhumane and rough way to treat with your body. Although people blame their bodies for their unruly appetites, overeating comes from the mind, not the body. Overeating happens when people are out of touch with their appetite. A slower approach to eating is more respectful of your body.

Sometimes modern food fails to satisfy your appetite. After several days working hard on a home improvement project, I realized I couldn't eat enough to satisfy myself. Nothing would tame my appetite, no matter how much I kept eating. At first I thought I was eating more because of the physical labor. But soon I realized I was eating more because my diet was depleted of much needed nutrients and minerals. I was working long hours and living on empty carbs. I hadn't eaten any greens in days. My body didn't need more calories; it was hungry for vitamins and minerals.

When you are nutrient deficient, your appetite tells you to keep eating food, any food, until your body gets what it needs. You will still feel hungry, even if you've already eaten a large amount of food. Refined foods and foods that are processed or precooked at the factory, like potato chips and white bread, often lack nutrients and minerals. Your body, built to survive in a natural environment, doesn't realize that these foods will never and could never fulfil its nutritional requirements. So it tells you to eat another potato chip, searching the haystack of food for the needle of nutritional satisfaction.

Many people overeat because they are nutrient and mineral deficient despite their high caloric intake. This leads to weight gain and feeling as if they have an unruly appetite that cannot be tamed. You may feel like you are trying to fill a hollow leg, but the emptiness isn't in the quantity of food. It's the quality. Poor quality food makes you hungrier. Your body tries its best to help you get the nutrition it needs to function well, but if you feed it empty calories, you will feel unsatisfied and starved.

Even if you've eaten plenty of vitamins and minerals, you may be hungry because your diet is missing a specific macronutrient (carbohydrate, fat, or protein). People on low-fat diets often crave carbohydrates to make up the difference. People on low-carbohydrate diets often feel irresistibly drawn to binge on cookies or sweets. An especially common case is protein deficiency. Nine times out of ten, unruly sugar cravings are really a protein deficiency in disguise, a fact that every vegetarian is familiar with. This is because one of the main functions of protein is helping you regulate blood sugar levels. If you are low on proteins, your blood sugar levels will be unstable, making you crave sweets. When you are low on proteins you'll keep eating and eating yet nothing will seem to satisfy you. If you struggle with sugar cravings, try adding more protein to your diet and see if that reduces your sugar cravings. Instead of following a low-fat diet, or a low carb diet, at Joyful Belly we recommend you simply eat a balanced diet, and let nature take care of the rest.

Many people eat nutrient poor food because they feel like they can't afford higher quality, nutrient-rich food. However, organic carrots, potatoes, beans, and frozen food are only 20% more expensive than conventionally grown food. If 20% seems like it will break your budget, consider how these foods will satisfy your appetite sooner because of their high nutrient density. You might even end up saving money by eating less! Recent studies have created some controversy whether organic product contains higher nutrient density, but at Joyful Belly we believe that difference in taste is proof of the difference. If you can't afford organic foods, whole foods like brown rice, beans, and fruits have more nutrients than processed foods like bread, juices, and tortillas. They may seem more expensive in the moment, but in the long-term these options aren't just healthier, they are also more efficient because they satisfy you with less food.

Cultural beliefs can distort your appetite. In my Italian American family, the generosity of the host may be measured by the generosity of the portions on the table. Large quantities of food create an atmosphere of hospitality, warmth, & success. The worries of poverty feel far away at a full table of steaming, heaping food. Large American portions serve as a sign of our confidence and strength as a culture. The Supersize Me™ mentality taps deeply into the American Dream. The priorities of this dream can supersede your capacity to eat.

Your appetite may also be misled by the portion on your plate. This is an example of the popular saying, "the eyes are bigger than the stomach." It is undeniable that portions in the United States have gotten out of hand. Recently, when walking into Sam's Club, I saw humongous muffins that were 3 times the size of a normal muffin. This mutant muffin was enough to feed a person for the whole day. Armed with one of these muffins, you could inadvertently forget to notice its size and consume the whole muffin in one sitting, especially if you were distracted talking to a friend or perhaps in front of the TV. Distraction also distorts appetite, mostly because you don't even notice what you're eating or when you are full!

Even the size of plates, bowls, and serving dishes can distort your appetite. The size of serving ware has grown exponentially. And with it, portion size has too. Smaller bowls, plates, and platters can help each of us to return to the humility of ancestral portions in our own way. Smaller bowls, plates, and platters encourage slower eating and appreciation of the food as well, because every bite matters.

Portions have a way of becoming habits. Each time you eat, your stomach gets used to eating more. Your stomach expects you to eat more next time as well. It may take some time, but the more you can bring awareness to your stomach's sense of satisfaction, the easier it will be for you to stop when you are truly full as opposed to judging your appetite by the size of your plate. A good rule of thumb to prevent overeating is to remember to always leave space in your stomach. A bit of space gives your stomach room to churn and mix the food with digestive juices. If you have put so much food in your stomach that you are overstuffed, the food will squeeze out the other end, damaging the small intestine. It can also distend your stomach, causing loss of stomach function.

How much space should you leave in your stomach for digestion? Ayurveda says to fill your stomach ⅓ with food, ⅓ with fluid, and ⅓ with air for optimal digestion. This means eating until your stomach is ⅔ full (⅓ with food and ⅓ with fluid) and then pausing to check in and see how you feel. It can be a sheer act of faith to stop eating when your stomach isn't full yet. Rest assured though, within a half hour, as your blood sugar starts to rise, you will feel satisfied, light, and energetic.

An odd routine can distort your appetite. If you schedule lunch at odd hours because of a demanding work schedule or a social engagement, your appetite may not be ready yet for a meal. Then you will have to force the food down even though you aren't very hungry. Eating together is a wonderful thing to do for health and happiness, but not everybody gets hungry at the same time. One person's appetite may not be ready yet. If your work or social situation forces you to eat at times when your appetite is lacking, order light options from the menu. Light, easy to digest options won't disturb your system too much. A salad, a few vegetable sides, or even a simple tea are all fine, light options. Do your best to avoid overeating when you aren't hungry (which is more common than you think!).

Stressful lifestyle habits, such as rushing through the day with an agitated mind, compromises your ability to pay attention to food cravings, make healthy choices, and listen to your appetite. Many people make impulsive choices about food because they are rushing, or simply want to fill their belly quickly and easily. You may feel like you do not have the time to make a healthy food choice, or are too overwhelmed to think or to figure out what to eat. This can lead to overeating. But if you are stressed out and overwhelmed, you'll first need to create some mental space, and give yourself permission to slow down for a minute. It only takes 30 seconds or less to pay attention to your body and sort through your cravings. Taking this time to select the right foods can help reduce your portion sizes, truly satisfy your cravings, and will bring myriad other rewards as well.

You can evade your appetite limitations and warning signals by eating too quickly. In the United States people eat too fast. We don't spend enough time enjoying our food. The French spend an average of 2 hours a day eating meals. How does that compare with the time you take for meals? An average fast food meal, for instance, takes only 10 minutes to eat, down to 8 minutes in a workplace cafeteria. Children at school spend only 7.3 minutes eating their lunch and that's simply too fast.[3]

Consider what happens when you eat a meal too quickly. As you can imagine, your appetite would hardly have time to catch up before you had already wolfed down the entire meal. Your body is actually designed to eat very slowly. Your hunger diminishes and satisfaction increases slowly while eating. It is essential that you allow your body the time it needs to communicate with you and abate your appetite. The feedback loop takes time. Your body needs enough time to start digesting the food before it can tell you whether you've eaten enough nutrients. Generally, you should take at least 20 minutes to finish a meal. If your body takes about 20 minutes to abate your appetite and you eat a meal in 10, you could ingest double

---

3 Jan Chozen Bays, *Mindful Eating* (Boston: Shambhala, 2009), 98.

the amount your body really wanted and needed. Rushing through meals is one way to confuse your appetite.

Have you ever had a fresh-baked chocolate chip cookie that tasted so good that you ate the whole thing so quickly that you barely even noticed it? The more someone likes a food, the faster they tend to eat it. When food is delicious people tend to eat as if they are afraid of some other person snatching it away. They want to eat as much of it as possible, but then it is gone all too fast and you are robbed of your enjoyment! You would think that if you really loved a food, you would want the experience to last as long as possible. If you really loved ice cream, you'd want to eat it slowly and enjoy it more. But that's not what happens. People tend to gobble up food that they love. As if in a trance, they eat so quickly that they completely miss out on the experience. Instead, make a commitment to savor delicious food, and enjoy the entertainment food provides. Amazing food can inspire you to overeat if you aren't careful.

Personally, I've found this tendency to overeat amazing food is only problematic when it is a processed food. When sugar & kids are involved, this tendency to hoard and devour is nothing short of devilish. I remember my daughter throwing a temper tantrum a few years ago when I cut her cupcake in half. She wanted the whole cupcake. No matter how much she's craving a carrot, she has never lost her temper over that!

Eating more slowly and cultivating a slower lifestyle is not only healthier, it will transform your experience of food into a pleasurable one. Just as your body feels unsatisfied with empty carbs, it will also feel unsatisfied if you are eating food that tastes bad. Many people deny themselves the pleasure of food in order to lose weight. It is this curious lack of enjoyment that, paradoxically, keeps you desperate for more satisfaction, causing you to eat more. Nothing increases portion size more than dissatisfaction. When you eat food that is truly enjoyable, you can find complete satisfaction in a tiny bite. Dissatisfaction distorts your appetite. At Joyful Belly, we spend a lot of time thinking about foods, mulling over which ingredients we might enjoy, and determining which foods feel good for a specific moment or season. These conversations are always enjoyable, entertaining, and fruitful.

The French eat more fat, the Italians more carbs, and the Germans more protein, all with less heart disease. After all the dietary comparisons between Europe, America, and other countries, it seems the only difference in America is the inhuman pace of eating, portion size, and relative social isolation. Europeans eat together, and spend more time eating. Europeans use mealtime to not only enjoy the experience of food more fully, but also to enjoy each other's company. The meal itself is a meaningful and sacred act for sharing with others and bonding. In America, so many people eat just because they are lonely. Too often Americans eat in front of the TV, in a rush on our lunch break, or even when we are fighting with our spouses. The mealtime lacks care, attention, and enjoyment. There is not enough time dedicated to enjoying, tasting, experiencing, and fully consuming every aspect of the food.

When I lived in Paris, I would eat out at restaurants often. I delighted in the attention given to food in France. They attended to the entire experience of eating, not only the taste. The food was fresh and flavorful. The environment was relaxed and pleasant. I was astonished to see the patrons at the restaurant quizzing the waiter about the food, including each ingredient and its exact preparation, as if they wanted to envision the entire meal before eating it. The customers wanted to speak directly with the chef, who was happy to oblige, and even eager to talk about his creative inspirations behind the meal. The waiters would seem disappointed if I didn't ask questions about the food. The chef would feel betrayed, after investing so much heartfelt passion in his art, as if the meal was unworthy of discussion. Such chefs and waiters are not so easily dismissed. They want to know that you are engaged with your meal, and appreciating the food. Discussing the food means you are paying attention and interested. That you are inspired by their creation. In such a restaurant, food is to be explored, a mystery to delve into, a gem to be discovered.

It became very exciting for the waiter and me to have this dynamic conversation, because we both loved food. And, it encouraged me to slow down and notice the food more. We would talk about the history of the sauces, or how a curious mélange of spices gave the compote a Middle Eastern flare. Or, I might as easily have complained that the olive oil was overcooked, to the point where this naturally sharp oil was rendered flavorless, and probably devoid of nutrients as well. I would study the menu at least a half an hour before deciding what to eat, giving me plenty of time to imagine the food in advance. These considerations can help you get in touch with your appetite too. Imagining the food beforehand not only helps you know how much you want to eat, but also helps you identify your cravings so you know what you want to eat. Your appetite is refined not only by choosing the right quantity, but also the right food, using taste and enjoyment as a guide.

By the time I left Paris, I had grown in the art of meal analysis. It suited my affinity for culinary perfection. I relished in the full attention and expression I could give to the art. Food exploration in French culture helped me discover the pleasure of food in a deeper way, to appreciate and discover subtleties in the satisfaction it would bring. To many, an adventure into the joy of eating might seem superfluous, or even an indulgence. But the joy of food is wholly rooted in biology. Honest food cravings are an authentic expression of your body's nutritional needs. You are made to enjoy food that is right for you. You can trust your body's desire as long as you are eating whole foods, minimally processed. The exploration of your cravings brings to conscious light the foods your body needs to be healthy. Appetite, after all, should lead to nourishment. The exploration of your cravings helps you efficiently satisfy your body's needs without overeating.

When I came back to the States, I invited my friends to continue this tradition. We would spend a half an hour discussing the menu options, which sauce would go well with which fish, and with which salad. We would get excited, "Oh, look how much ingenuity and creativity was in that recipe!" We tried to guess the intentions of the chef. What did he want us to experience when he invented the ensemble? Why did he add mango to the salsa sauce? What was the point of roasting the pears?

It was fun and surprising each time. Instead of wolfing it down as simply a means to survive, the meal became a ceremony, a ritual. Instead of getting on to the next thing, the meal itself became the focal point of entertainment for the day. Celebrating the meal helped me stay connected with my body, to my friends, and to the food.

There are many occasions where enjoying food as cuisine seems unwelcome and out of place. Once at TGI Fridays I tried to engage the waitress on the nuances of a thickened potato peel. She seemed unimpressed by my interest and annoyed. These kinds of establishments see food as fodder to fill the belly. The kind of food enjoyment they advertise is belly satisfaction instead of true satisfaction. Belly satisfaction is no doubt fun, but can be problematic if you are struggling with overeating. Start to notice when food advertisements are marketing belly satisfaction as opposed to true satisfaction, satisfaction that goes down to your bones, making you feel fresh and vital.

How often have you eaten a meal while engrossed in conversation, watching TV, or driving? Then, twenty minutes later you look down at your plate and all the food is gone. You may not have even tasted it. You may have forgotten to enjoy the food. Eating while distracted undermines your relationship with food. TV dinners, Hot Pockets, & meal replacement shakes subvert the all-important ceremony of selecting ingredients, preparing a meal, and eating. As you lose touch with the ceremony surrounding a meal, you also lose touch with your appetite and cravings. Your appetite can't serve its purpose well when you eat without paying attention.

Distraction could even cost you thousands of dollars. Not too long ago, my sister gave my mother and father a box of Oreo™ cookies. This special box of Oreo™ cookies had an announcement on the packaging of a contest to find the thousand dollar cookie. Along with the announcement was a picture of the winning Oreo™ cookie. This cookie had a unique design, different from the others. My father, who loves contests and finding hidden treasure, was excited to participate. While they were eating, there it was - they found the winning cookie! They were very excited about winning the prize. My mother immediately called my sister to give her the news. While she was talking to my sister over the phone, my mother kept munching on the plate of cookies. Soon she hung up the phone and my father asked her for the cookie. My mother looked down at the plate and all the cookies were gone! Including the special Oreo cookie with the winning design. My mother had eaten the cookie! Ayurveda says never to eat while distracted. You could miss out on the prize, literally!

Instead, reconnect with your appetite by actually tasting the food. Overcome the epidemic of distraction and realize that as exciting as the evening news is, what's on your plate is equally exciting. There is something wonderful about food. Don't miss it. Think of it as exploration and adventure. Be curious about your food. Be in awe. Be in wonder about the food. How can this spinach taste so good? What are all the flavors in this sauce? What does it remind me of? Let yourself celebrate and appreciate food. Then you will be aware and synchronized with your appetite.

It is hard to do. I know it is a challenge. Today, even though I preach the practice of eating with awareness, I sometimes get distracted during the meal and forget to enjoy it. I always feel like I missed out on something important and joyful - all the while hurting my body by putting things in it without even noticing. Slowing down and taking the time to enjoy your food may be a struggle for you. But over time, you start to appreciate the benefits, both in terms of quality of life and also efficiency.

If you don't know how to turn your meal into a ceremony, start by giving thanks, which is one of the best ways to introduce some time and patience into the process of eating. Giving thanks forces you to stop whatever you are doing. When you give thanks you turn off the TV, stop talking, put your fork down, and pause. In that pause you can say thank you in a heartfelt way, to God, the cook, the farmer, and others for their efforts on your behalf, appreciating all that was accomplished to bring you this plate of food. Appreciation not only improves the joy of eating; in that pause, you also create an opportunity to reconnect to your appetite and how you are feeling. You can remember to appreciate the food as a gift. You can set an intention for how you want to enjoy the moment and enjoy the food.

I have always loved the term, "Saying Grace" as it applies to thanking God and petitioning His blessing for a meal. In every other circumstance besides a meal, it's just called prayer. But when it comes to food, the sustenance of life, the prayer itself becomes a delicious act of grace. Whatever your belief system is - whatever God you give thanks to - reconnecting the act of eating to its sacred origins is essential to lift your awareness of food to a more subtle level, and inspire creativity. Who knows what inspiration you will discover in this brief moment?

After you have said grace, look at the food. You can look at its shape, its color, its texture, its heat, and its moisture. Ask yourself questions about the food. Look at the quantity of food on the platter and ask yourself, "How much do I need to eat to be comfortably full?" The

Ayurvedic way to extend your grace practice is to hold the plate up to your nose and smell it deeply. Inhale the scent of each item on your plate. If you close your eyes while smelling the food, your sense of smell will be sharper. You will really be able to tune into the food. If you have a serving of chicken, a serving of greens, and a serving of rice on your plate, smell each of them 3 times so that your body can start to decide which food it wants to eat and how much. Your interaction with the food, smelling, and tasting it, can cause radical shifts in dietary choices that seem contradictory, depending on the ever changing needs of your body.

When you consider the smell and taste of your food, your body may give you a surprising answer, one that seems irrational. One February, my daughter ate all the beans I could give her, when in the previous month I could hardly get her to eat a single one. Maybe you are craving different foods from last month too? There may be a difference in the season, or in your body's nutritional needs that causes this shift. Kids seem to get obsessed about some particular food for several weeks, wanting to eat the same food over and over again. Then, just as suddenly, they have an aversion to the very same food. The act of smelling the food brings you into the present moment and invites your body to participate in your food choices. The interaction with your food that smelling brings will help you sharpen your awareness of your appetite.

Once you've said grace and smelled your food, continue the ceremony by taking a bite. You can take the first bite with your eyes closed. Try to get as much sensation from the first bite as possible. Put the spoon or fork down so that you are not anticipating the second bite and check in with yourself about what you are experiencing. Continue to chew the bite until the taste starts to fade, which will happen fairly quickly. After about ten to fifteen chews, the flavor starts to disappear. When the taste is gone and the food fully liquefied, that is your sign to swallow.

Once your mouth is empty, notice that sensation as well. How long can you detect the flavor after swallowing? Notice as many sensations as you can in your mouth. Does it feel tingly? Does it feel smooth or rough when you rub your tongue on the roof of your mouth? Does your mouth feel dry or wet? Does it feel warm or cool? Does it feel irritated? Where do you feel the experience? How is it different from previous experiences? Challenge yourself to write a whole poem or page in your journal about your experience. This might be a good time to take a sip of water and cleanse your mouth before the next bite. You can take a sip and swish it around your mouth just like a wine connoisseur would to clear his palate.

As you finish your first bite, notice when you have the impulse to pick the fork up again. You will feel the impulse arise naturally. Then take another bite. This time, notice the texture of the food while you are chewing. Is it soft or hard? Dense or fluffy? Crunchy or mushy? Rough or smooth? As you chew your second bite, notice what your tongue is doing in your mouth. It's almost like the leg of an octopus. Your tongue has a mind of its own. It probes the food, mulls and mingles with the food. The tongue has a special role in helping you experience food. The tongue wants to give you a complete taste experience.

Take a third bite. This time, notice the taste again. Does the food still taste as good? The taste of food actually changes with each bite. This is why paying attention can be fascinating. You can eat a banana and the taste of the banana in the beginning is very different than the taste of the banana at the end. Generally, taste changes every five bites. It seems to morph and change with time - and it's really not the banana that is changing, but it is actually *you* that is changing. A banana might taste amazing after the first bite but may bore you by the end. You don't notice the change in flavor from bite to bite but you do notice after five bites or ten. The first bite of food is most stimulating and after that the taste begins to wane. If you aren't paying attention, you won't notice. If you don't notice you might as well be eating cardboard. I remember times in my life when I was truly thirsty. In those moments the taste of water was truly heavenly. If you have been working outside in the hot sun and you have been sweating, that glass of water refreshes your whole being. You can almost see it sparkling in the sunshine. There is something uplifting about it because it is satisfying a deep need.

As you continue through your meal ask the people around you, "How do you like the food? How does it taste to you? Is it hitting the spot?" Your friend might reply, "The food was heavenly." If the food hits the spot, you know that it was heavenly food - manna from heaven. Then ask, "What flavors did you notice in the food?", "What about the texture?", "What is it about the food that most appeals to you?" Consult your friends and make the food a bonding experience - engage the people around you. It often makes the experience of food even richer.

Remembering and recognizing your experiences of eating food is a joyful way to regulate your appetite. There are so many ways that your appetite may be fooled, distorted, eluded, or ignored, too many to mention in this book. However, by eating slowly, with ceremony and appreciation, you will start to notice how you have been overriding your body's signs and signals. You'll start to reconnect to your biological cues again. You will start to become a connoisseur of food and an expert on your body's relationship with food. With your active curiosity, you will soon find many more ways to listen to your body. As you do, you will notice that you make healthier choices and eat healthier portions naturally.

Chapter 4: Taste & Food Cravings

*

In Ayurveda, the tongue is a valuable diagnostic tool. In our clinic, people often feel shy when we ask to see their tongue. But when we ask clients, they feel embarrassed and exposed, as if by showing their tongue they are showing a very private part of their body. Ayurveda, along with many healing traditions, affirms the revealing nature of the tongue. Because it tells such an important story about you and your health, you may feel vulnerable showing your tongue. If you have a bad taste on your tongue or an unsightly coating, you might even feel ashamed about your tongue.

However the tongue is an important organ that you cannot ignore, especially when it comes to weight loss. It is a map of your health and imbalances, and the key to understanding your food cravings. When you understand the tongue, and the tastes on it, you learn about yourself and your imbalances. While scientists in white lab coats use machines to test the nutritional properties of food, as an individual you use your tongue to sample the taste of food. Your tongue is the instrument of your personal food laboratory, an essential tool in the process of making good food choices. Many people make food decisions from memory without checking their tongue. They ignore the food laboratory in their mouth. They return to a restaurant and order the same sandwich, time after time, without taking a fresh perspective on what they truly want.

To harness the expert nutritional wisdom of the tongue is simple enough: start with taste. Many people think taste is epicurean only - that taste buds exist for your delight. On the contrary, every taste sensation is full of meaning and significance. In Ayurveda, you learn what to eat from taste and experience, not from a book. It's tempting to think that someone else has the answers, that someone else knows better than you do. Books certainly contain valuable information about nutrition. There's a comfort to letting someone else be your leader. But only you and your body know what nutrients you actually need, right now. In Western Medicine, the pharmaceutical benefits of food are determined by statistical analysis. But in Ayurveda your relationship with food is more personal and unique. A book can't know whether you've been sweating excessively, or haven't eaten enough greens lately, or have other unique nutritional deficiencies. Instead, by examining your cravings and tasting your food very *very* carefully, your body will tell you what it wants to eat.

Diligently note how the food makes you feel over the next several hours. You might feel refreshed after drinking lemonade. Giddy after a glass of wine. You might feel hearty and strong after eating roast beef. Or, you might feel sedated after a bowl of mashed potatoes. In Ayurveda, these feelings are the medicinal effects of the food, which are used pharmacologically. When you practice Ayurveda, the experiences you have after eating food are also the 'nourishment' you get from food. Each time you figure out how a certain food makes you feel, you have acquired a new tool which can be used medicinally. You can eat those same foods anytime you want to recreate the feeling. Anytime you want to be refreshed again, have another glass of lemonade.

Taste helps you identify the food that will bring the effects you want. By tasting and experiencing you will be able to pinpoint exactly what your body wants and needs moment to moment. You simply taste your food and listen to your body. Over time you'll know exactly how to select the right food for the experiences you want. That's why enjoying your food isn't just entertainment, it's also the path to health.

You might find that some unhealthy food choices seem to 'taste good' initially, but after further consideration of the effects, they aren't as good. Your palate becomes more discerning. When you notice how poorly it makes you feel, suddenly the taste isn't so appealing. If you have ever gotten sick and vomited after eating something, you'll never want to eat that food again. The next time you have the food, you may notice that it disgusts you rather than pleases your tongue. Similarly, by paying attention to how you feel after eating, your tongue will learn what it likes.

Similarly, just because you liked the taste of apples a few weeks ago, that doesn't mean you will like them this week as well. Your tongue, the tastes on it, and your food cravings are always changing, with the seasons, with the weather, and as your body changes with age. When I was a child, candy tasted really good to me, but as an adult, I have lost my taste for it. It is not that the candy changed, it is that I have changed. Generally your cravings change every 3 weeks as the season changes. An illness can also distort your taste and cravings. As you and the environment around you changes, your body must adapt, especially in the area of diet. In the summer, a hearty pot roast is not as appealing as a fruit smoothie. Your taste buds and food preferences adapt to these changes in your body. Food literally tastes different as the seasons change.

Note that it is the taste of the food, not the flavor, that changes. There is a big difference between taste and flavor. Flavor comes from the smell of the banana, and is unique to a banana. Taste is much more general. It is what you experience if you hold your nose shut while eating. Each food has a unique combination of sweet, sour, salty, bitter, astringent, and pungent tastes. The flavor of the soda doesn't change no matter how much you drink it. Only the taste changes.

Another funny thing is that the more food you eat with a particular taste, the less you can taste it. Tastes missing from your diet taste stronger, while tastes that are abundant in your diet taste weaker. In this way, your own diet can distort your natural taste experience and even your appetite. If your blood is already really sweet from eating lots of sugary foods, soda won't taste very sweet at all. It will just taste bland. Then you may feel unsatisfied, and add more and more sugar to make the beverage "sweet enough" for your taste buds. Paradoxically, it's not the soda that isn't sweet enough but rather your blood that is too sweet to detect the natural sweetness in the soda. This is why people with hyperglycemia have a high tolerance for sweet taste.

If you put something sour in your mouth, like a lemon, it won't even taste very sour if your body is already too sour. But if lemons taste very sour to you, you are probably missing sours in your diet. When you haven't eaten anything sour in a while, the lemon will taste very strong. If you eat 5 wedges of lemon in a row, you'll notice that the 5th slice doesn't taste as sour as the first one.

If you absolutely hate the taste of simple bitter greens like kale, iceberg lettuce, endives, and arugula, that is a sign that bitters are missing from your diet. Many of our clients absolutely hate the taste of bitters, so they never eat greens. This is not really because their body doesn't like bitters, but because they are missing bitters from their diet. You can teach your tongue to enjoy bitters again by eating them daily. As you reintroduce bitters into your diet, you'll notice within 40 days that bitter greens and vegetables are more palatable and less intense tasting.

What does all this mean? If the taste of a banana can change from the top of the banana to the bottom of the banana, or if the intensity of bitter taste can change after 40 days of eating bitters, it means that taste is not in the food but on your tongue. The tastes you experience when you eat a banana show your relationship to the banana. Taste is not just about what you're eating, but your body's relationship to what you're eating. And that's ever-changing and ever-shifting, which is why paying attention is so critical to knowing what your body wants and what your body needs.

Once your body has had enough of a taste, it is like having enough of a nutrient. That's because your body uses taste to guess which nutrients are in the food. Instead of counting calories, proteins, and minerals, your body measures your experience of food, starting with taste and the tongue. As your nutritional needs are satisfied, the taste of your food changes. If you eat enough carbs, naturally you won't be hungry for carbs. If you eat enough protein, you won't want any more protein-rich foods. Similarly with taste, if you eat enough sour, sour will seem bland and uninteresting. When you have satisfied one of your taste cravings - sweet, sour, salty, pungent, bitter, or astringent - it loses its flavor and appeal. You may not know which minerals are in the foods you are eating, yet taste remains a crude yardstick to measure your nutritional needs. Taste and your tongue have adequately served mankind for millions of years and are thus exceptionally reliable, when exposed to natural rather than processed foods.

Have you ever tried to taste your tongue with nothing in your mouth? Simply rub your tongue against the top of your mouth while it is empty, and notice. What taste did you find? What is the texture of your saliva? What else did you notice? As Ayurvedic practitioners, we check the taste of the tongue several times throughout the day. Monitoring the ever-changing tastes on your tongue helps you stay attuned to the needs of your body in ways that we will explain later. What you taste on your tongue is really the taste of your saliva. When the taste on your tongue changes, it means your saliva is changing, which also means your blood is changing. When you know your taste, you know your blood. The composition of saliva reflects the composition of your blood. In Ayurveda we say that the taste of your saliva is the taste of your blood.

Your tongue is constantly reading your blood and triggering desire for the foods you need most, at this moment in time. As often as your blood chemistry changes, the urges of your tongue and the foods you crave will change. If your blood sugar drops and you feel shaky, you will naturally crave sugar to bring it back up. Cravings are always changing. Your tongue may even seem capricious if it is doing its job right. Once you realize that your food preferences change as your blood and taste change, you start to realize that your food cravings aren't merely whimsical. Instead, changes in your food preferences are an outcome of changes happening deeper within. Taste becomes a very rich diagnostic tool, telling you about your blood and things that are happening internally in your body. By assessing the taste in your mouth, you know how much toxins are in your blood, your blood sugar levels, the quality of your circulation, and many other imbalances.

Your tongue is designed to help you choose healthy foods. Ultimately, the tongue is the brain behind all your food cravings. Your tongue translates your blood chemistry into an impulse, an urge for a certain type of food. In other words, your tongue translates chemistry into cravings. It helps you by reading the needs of your body, based on a sample of saliva, and creating a taste craving. In this way, your tongue guides your body's food preferences. The whole purpose and reason for the evolution of taste is to prevent you from eating unhealthy foods, and guide you to healthy food choices for your particular body type. If your circulation is sluggish, for example, you'll naturally crave stimulating, warm, bitter foods. In an ideal world, your tongue should take pleasure in what is healthy for you, while harmful food should seem distasteful. Sometimes the accuracy of your taste buds becomes perverted, especially if you're not in the habit of listening to your cravings or if there are toxins in your body. Your tongue might crave foods that will actually imbalance you more, rather than less.

Checking the taste on your tongue is a very personal way to get to know your body and monitor your health. Everyone has a unique taste in their mouth, and it's a moving target. Your saliva may have a sweet, bitter, sour, or salty taste. Perhaps your palate is moist, or maybe it's dry. Once you know the taste on your tongue, you'll naturally want to know, "what does the taste mean?" Don't worry about the answer yet; just start by noticing. You can do it now as you read. Even if you can't describe your experience intellectually, checking your tongue throughout the day will develop your intuition and keep you tuned into your body.

So what is the taste of your blood? If you have a sweet taste in your mouth, maybe your blood sugar levels are high? If you have a sour taste, maybe you have acid reflux? If the taste on your tongue is salty, maybe you are retaining water? If the taste on your tongue is bitter, perhaps your liver is stressed? If the taste is astringent and dry, maybe you are dehydrated? If your mouth feels irritated (pungent), maybe you have inflammation in your GI tract?

As the tastes on your tongue change with the chemistry of your bodily fluids, so does the appearance of your tongue. In Ayurveda, a coating on the tongue is a sign of toxic build-up called *ama* in the body. If you have a yucky coating or taste on your tongue, this is an important symptom to address and fix. If you want to improve your health and lose weight, you must minimize the coating because most likely these toxins are depressing your metabolism and clogging up your circulation. Refreshing your palate with gum or breath mints may provide a short term Band-Aid to the yuckiness on your tongue, but it doesn't fix the imbalance in your blood which is causing the bad taste. You must address the yuckiness at the root level.

The good news is that you can repair a yucky tongue without too much trouble. Simply eat light, easily digestible foods for several days. The famous Ayurvedic rice and bean dish called 'kitchari' is a satisfying way to cleanse and remove a coating on the tongue naturally. You can also sip CCF tea (cumin coriander and fennel tea) throughout the day during your cleanse and take triphala at night. CCF tea is a simple tea brewed with equal parts cumin, coriander, and fennel. You can make it yourself at home, or buy it online. Triphala is a famous Ayurvedic herbal formula you can also purchase. A few days of this light and simple fare, together with these herbal teas, can help your metabolism to improve, your blood sugar to stabilize, and your body to eliminate toxins. This won't work for everyone, but it does for most people. After a few days, you will notice the coating on your tongue retreating further and further back on the tongue. By the end of the cleanse, the coating may be totally gone!

The more you pay attention to your tongue and the tastes on it, the more you will start to notice the many ways food affects your tongue. You will notice the favorable taste that certain foods leave on your tongue and the yucky taste that others leave. If food leaves a yucky taste, it is unhealthy for you. From there, you can discern which foods are going to balance you versus which foods will create imbalance. Then, you will participate consciously in choosing foods that will fix the taste on your tongue. Along the way, you'll fix the imbalances in your blood, and enjoy a renewed fresh and vital feeling - just by following the taste on your tongue.

As you explore the relationship between taste and healthy food choices, you'll notice that for most foods, the effect the food has on your body corresponds to the taste in the food. Each of the six tastes in food has certain healing properties. Two foods with the same taste, though perhaps radically different in other ways, often have similar medicinal effects. Your tongue is designed to help you choose those tastes whose medicinal effects that are the right matches for your Sweet foods build body mass, which some people need. Sweet taste will also make you more compassionate and sweet emotionally, though perhaps lethargic. It will also give you quick energy, but may make you tired and depressed later. Most foods that taste sweet have these effects. When you know that, you can consciously choose how much sweet taste to include in your diet.

Sour food tends to stimulate secretions, stimulate energy, increase moisture, flush glands, and move fluids. Some people already have a lot of moisture and sourness in their body. They might have sweaty palms and feel like their mood is sour. In that case, your tongue probably won't want foods with more of a sour effect. Other people need the stimulating properties of sour because they have a low appetite due to dryness in their digestive tract, or are too scattered because of dryness in the kidneys.

Salty foods make you retain water. They also increase your desire. Salt nourishes and strengthens nerves, which makes you feel paradoxically stimulated and grounded at the same time. Spicy or pungent foods irritate your tissues and increase your heart rate. They add pizzazz, and can "spice up your life" when you feel bored. Spicy foods lead to hot or fiery emotions. Astringent foods tighten up tissues that are lax or flabby, which may be helpful if your skin or muscles lack tone. Astringent foods cool inflammation. Bitter foods create a feeling of lightness and clarity, including mental clarity. Too many bitter foods can make you feel critical, austere, and disappointed. Each taste has many more properties than those listed here. Ayurveda studies taste in great depth and you can find many more effects of sweet, sour, salty, pungent, astringent, and bitter tastes in introductory Ayurvedic sources.

Although we talk about foods as having sweet, sour, salty, pungent, bitter or astringent tastes, the real taste of a food is the effect it has on your body. If food makes you feel drowsy, that is the true taste of the food. For all practical purposes, you could say that the food tastes "drowsy." You could also say this is the taste of the food at a cellular level. The taste you experience on your tongue is merely an approximation of the real taste. The tongue uses taste to predict the real effects of the food you are eating and is somewhat accurate at predicting the effects of most natural foods.

You can develop your skill in predicting how food will interact with your body. Just like any skill, practice makes perfect. If you want to be fit and athletic, it helps to work out in order to develop that capacity in your body. If you want to be smarter, it helps to read books to increase the capacity of your brain. If you want to know how different foods affect your body and how to heal with food, you have to practice with different foods. Take a trip to a nearby farmer's market, or health food store. Browse the produce aisle utilizing as many of your five senses as possible to find something appealing. Ask yourself, does the food smell 'tasty'? Does it look tasty? When you eat the food, savor the experience. Pay close attention to how you feel after eating, and remember the taste. The more you spend time practicing, the more you will understand your relationship to food. As you start to understand the relationship between taste and effect, you can start to predict consciously how certain foods will make you feel with a single bite!

If your tongue has been tricked by processed foods, distorted by toxins, habits, taste memories, or even distractions while eating, it will fail to guide you correctly and you may end up eating food that is harmful to you. Many processed foods are specifically designed to circumvent your body's natural awareness and intelligence of taste. The accuracy of your tongue and all five senses is very important to your health. If your taste buds have been distorted, you can enhance the accuracy of your taste buds by eating natural foods and through gentle cleansing (such as the kitchari cleanse mentioned above). That way you can make sure you know what you are eating and won't be fooled by processed foods!

Some food seems to taste good in the moment, like ice cream and donuts. But then, ten minutes later, you notice a bad taste in your mouth. Or sometimes after particularly offensive food, your mouth feels slimy, or maybe you feel tired and sluggish for the rest of the day. These are signs that your tongue failed to predict the effects and true nature of what you've eaten. If food tasted good but makes you feel bad later it means your cravings were misguided. If you frequently crave foods that leave a bad aftertaste, or that makes you feel bad or aggravates your symptoms, it means your tongue isn't accurately perceiving the taste, or you are not paying close enough attention to the this relationship between taste and effect.

Food mistakes such as this (and their aftermath) help us realize that our food choices matter and affect our health. Try not to be too hard on yourself for making these types of mistakes. We all make mistakes like this at times. Instead of berating yourself, spend a few minutes really paying attention to and noticing the way you feel after that food. If you can remember the feeling, you'll be less likely to make the same mistake in the future.

Ideally, if a bad aftertaste arises on your tongue after eating ice cream, the ice cream should taste just as foul as the result. A friend of mine ate brownies one night because she thought they looked and tasted so good. The next day she had a lot of diarrhea from the brownies. Her tongue, which told her that brownies were just about the best thing that ever happened to her, made a mistake. Clearly the taste of the brownies was better than the effect of the brownie. All that glitters is not gold and the tongue is easily fooled, especially by refined foods like the sugar and flour that went into the brownie. So my friend felt guilty for eating the brownie, when she really just needed to learn from the experience and re-educate her tongue. In these circumstances, instead of feeling guilty for a poor food choice, make an effort to remember the taste of the brownie and how it felt afterwards. In this case, a gooey, chocolate brownie caused indigestion and loose stools for my friend. By reconnecting the taste of the brownies to the effect, you will find it easier to make healthier food choices next time.

In addition to noticing and remembering the taste of those brownies and their effects, when you eat something that makes you feel good, remember the taste of that also. You might find yourself craving that food more often because you remember that it made you feel more awake, more energized, and lighter. Likewise, as you pay attention to the taste of food that makes you feel badly, you might find your cravings for them grow less and less over time. Ultimately, through this process of trial and error, you can refine your palette through experience. You will find you have an ability to change what's attractive to you just by noticing.

How will you know when your intuition is guiding you towards truly healthy foods, and when it has been hijacked by unruly food cravings? First, take a breath. Your capacity to discern what is good for you is incredibly important in all walks of life, not just with food. Think about all the trial and error each and every one of us experiences in navigating romantic and familial relationships. People come to understand the gift of true love through much suffering. As with relationships, recognize that discernment with food is the stuff of spiritual mastery. You may never reach the perfection of mind/body/spirit unity that would allow you to discern everything in your life to perfection. But you can hope, pray, and dedicate yourself to personal growth in choosing what is truly best for you and your community.

I once gave a lecture urging my weight-loss students not to eat late at night. That night one of the women in class succumbed to her food cravings (as we all do occasionally) and ate a heavy meal around 10pm. Eating late at night was a habit for her. That night after the lecture, for the first time, she truly noticed how short the enjoyment of the meal lasted and how physically badly she felt soon after and the next day. By the simple of act of noticing, without berating herself her desires and cravings began to change. It first started to affect the foods she chose. Then it started to affect the time of day she craved things. Eventually she no longer craved heavy foods at night regularly. And when she did, she was able to address the underlying emotional need instead of using food to soothe herself.

Sometimes your tongue says, "I want a piece of cheesecake." But that's not the tongue. That's the mind. The tongue is non-specific and perhaps a bit vague. You tongue wants you to eat a certain style or type of food. It might be in the 'mood' for something heavy. Or something sweet. These moods are very important in Ayurveda, so you should pay attention to them closely. What is your food mood right now? Is your tongue communicating with you and, if so, what is it saying? Once you know your food mood, you can figure out what to eat. The food moods of your tongue are usually a combination of tastes, textures, stimulation, and hydration.

Knowing that you want a piece of cheesecake is valuable information that can help you discover your food mood. You can ask yourself, "Why do I want this piece of cake? What will it do for me?" Cheesecake is heavy, sweet, and sour. It is filling, satisfying, and sedating. After a hearty slice of cheesecake, one can imagine drifting off into an easy night's sleep. If you've been feeling anxious or irritable, a thick slice of cheesecake provides that calm, relaxed mind you've been craving all day long. Your craving for comfort is not a bad craving. However, eating cheesecake to get the comfort you're craving can have unwanted side effects. Cheesecake is very rich and hearty. In excess, it could lead to weight gain. Instead, try to find a remedy that will help you feel comfortable and relaxed, without the side effects of cheesecake. For example, choose foods that are lighter than cheesecake but still satisfying and sweet - things like baked sweet potatoes or warm almond milk. Or, simply take a short walk in a pleasant natural setting. Find the comfort you need by reaching out to a loved one, or write in a journal. Once you know your food mood, you realize you have many options to fulfill your desires.

Let's follow that train of thought. Carla has had a hard and demanding week at work and is experiencing conflict with a co-worker. Friday while on her lunch break she thinks, "I really want a piece of cheesecake." However, if she were to notice more closely, she might find that what she really wants is something oily and heavy. If she were to delve into her craving for heavy food further, she might also notice that what she really wants is comfort and something to soothe the restless anxiety in the pit of her stomach. Her mind translates all of those things she craves - heavy, soothing, comforting, relaxing - into the quick fix of cheesecake. But really she arrived at this craving through a multi-layered process.

Somehow, your body knows that the cheesecake will be comforting and satisfying. You might not realize this association because it happens on a very subconscious level. A vision of cheesecake pops into your head and you just think you want cheesecake. If you are not aware of the food mood behind the craving, you might feel a bit out of control, and powerless to resist the compelling thought of eating a cheesecake.

When you become conscious of the process from emotions to food cravings, then you will know what really needs to be fixed. You will know the root of your craving. You know what your body really wants to feel stable, balanced, and happy. That is your true hunger and food craving. You could feed your body cheesecake, but your problems will return again. Or, you could wind down by going for a walk, by taking a few deep breaths, by saying a prayer, or by meditating. Or, you could simply buy yourself some flowers for the dining room table. Then, suddenly, the craving for cheesecake disappears, and you've avoided some potentially nasty side effects.

It's important to remember that cheesecake isn't a 'bad food.' For some people and on some occasions, it can be a healthy choice. Cheesecake may seem to relax you at first, but if your blood is already too rich it will make you feel depressed later. After the sugar crash is over, you'll find cheesecake actually exacerbates the anxiety you were trying to get rid of in the first place. That's why, as Thomas Jefferson wrote, "Do not bite at the bait of pleasure till you know there is no hook beneath it." Similarly, if you are trying to lose weight, cheesecake won't be the best home remedy for anxiety. You don't need to berate yourself for eating cheesecake, just pay attention to how it makes you really feel.

Sometimes people eat food not for comfort, but because they are bored. Each and everyone one of us wants to enjoy all the beautiful gifts of being alive. On its own, that desire is very beautiful and sacred. However, all too often the desire for abundance seems to degenerate into an addiction to stimulation. The tongue is very guilty of this, perhaps more so than other organs. The tongue is an organ of desire. Think about ketchup. Tartar sauce. Relish. Pickles. These foods delight the tongue and stimulate you. When we feel separate from the joyful celebration of life, food is an easy way to self-stimulate. What do you do when you're bored? If you're like me and everyone else I know, when life feels empty you open the fridge. Any kind of stimulation gratifies the tongue and seems to whisk boredom away.

My daughter is actually a great teacher of this. There's an outdoor cafe in Asheville that we frequent on summer evenings to enjoy a ginger beer. Ginger beer is a beverage just like root beer but with ginger instead. I remember the first time I gave my daughter a taste, when she was one and a half years old. She got a little frightened because it was fizzy and had a sharp taste but then she wanted more. And she loves that taste to this day, and often asks me to go to the cafe to get a ginger beer. It is fun when the tongue is stimulated, and it is even addicting. The fizziness on your tongue actually hurts if you take the time to notice it, but most people also like it. Everyone wants a party in their mouth, all the time. Wouldn't that be wonderful, if you could go through life with a party in your mouth all day long? Those intense taste experiences are very gratifying, very pleasurable, and you can easily get addicted to them. That's why it is important to discover when your tongue is craving a taste for a healthy reason, or if it is just searching for stimulation.

Through analyzing your food cravings and the emotions behind them in this manner, you come to understand how food, taste, blood chemistry and your emotions are connected. Then you are one step closer to understanding the nature of your cravings, and how your tongue is translating your blood chemistry into impulses. Figuring out your food moods is thus very important to figuring out the causes of your food cravings. The following is an example of how one person might approach their craving for ice-cream to think of ways they can satisfy those cravings healthfully:

Example: ICE CREAM

Q: What about ice-cream are you craving?

1) Are you actually craving something **Creamy**? You might be seeking emotional comfort, a way to alleviate insecurities, or perhaps you have some kind of inflammation you are trying to soothe. Instead, try a banana smoothie. It is also creamy, gooey, and sweet just like ice-cream, but much lighter.

2) Are you craving ice-cream because you want something **Cold**? Try a refreshing, cool glass of water. You might have internal heat; it may just be summertime and hot outside. Mint & other aromatic herbs can purge heat from your system. Lemonade is also a good option because it opens your pores. Bitter taste can cool you down, as can cilantro and cabbage juice.

3) Are you craving ice-cream because you want **Comfort**? Comfort foods tend to be high in calories. Instead, try a warm bowl of mashed sweet potatoes; or a hot bowl of chili. Sweet potatoes are a classic, healthy comfort food. Beans are heavy and comforting, but are very low in calories.

4) Are you craving ice-cream because you want **Oily**? Oily foods tend to be satisfying and hearty. They create a feeling of security and strength but are also high in calories. Instead, slice open an avocado and add a little bit of salt and black

pepper to it. It contains healthy fats and comes from nature.

5) Are you craving ice-cream because your body needs **Calcium**? If it's the chalkiness of ice-cream that you want, have a kale and tahini salad instead. Both sesame seeds and kale have more calcium than milk.

6) Are you craving ice-cream because you want something **Sweet?** Cravings for sweet taste commonly indicate a protein deficiency. Have you eaten any protein lately? Adding some heavy protein like meat might help, or beans and nuts if you are a vegetarian. It may also be a sign of low metabolism, or that you are tired and in an energy slump. Adding spices to your meals like ginger, cumin, and black pepper can all give metabolism a boost. Exercise is also going to be key, along with adding more bitter taste through greens and even *Tikta Ghrita* (bitter ghee) can help.

7) Are you craving ice-cream because you want something **Crunchy**? Sometimes the crunch of chocolate chips and an ice-cream cone feels very appealing. Crunchy cravings often mean your body is feeling congested and watery. In those instances, you may need some astringency through beans or pomegranate. Diuretics with insoluble fiber can be good too - things like celery or apples.

The Ayurvedic concept of taste isn't restricted to food alone. In conversation, people discuss their taste in art, in choosing a life partner, or in decorating a home.

You might believe a person has great artistic taste in area, but poor taste in another. On an esoteric level, the tongue is the organ responsible for these kinds of taste decisions as well. If you have good taste, it means your impulses are leading you to good choices. If you make decisions that lead to bad outcomes, it means you have poor taste. In Ayurveda, all disease begins with decisions and behaviors made in 'poor taste.'

For example, you might find a centerpiece for your table at the flea market that seems beautiful at the time and buy it for your home. But then, two weeks later, you lose interest in it and no longer like it. When that happens, it means you had poor taste. However, if you found one that was truly beautiful and you still enjoy it weeks and months and even years later, it was probably a decision made in good taste. In life, we always try to make good investments. We want to make choices that have enduring value.

Sometimes, like a wolf in sheep's clothing, food tricks your tongue. Or you realize later you shouldn't have bought the centerpiece. Or a person you trusted betrays you. The most insidious false tastes are when we betray ourselves, over and over again, by our own beliefs and worldview. Drinking too much alcohol to be social, or working too hard to improve your quality of life are examples of poor taste. If you are willing to humble yourself, you'll come to the painful realization that certain beliefs and attitudes that you're following haven't yielded the benefits you thought they would.

Since the tongue is responsible for taste decisions, for predicting the outcome of food and the outcome of your personal choices, on an esoteric level the tongue is also the physical organ of boundaries. If a person has good boundaries, they know how to draw the line in relationships. In the same way, the tongue is supposed to draw the line with food. A person with good boundaries usually has a strong tongue. You might know someone like this. Often, people with good boundaries enjoy a stable, secure home life. They are careful and discerning about who they let in their life and the foods they take into their body. Out of balance, a person with strong boundaries may be wary of change and feel stuck in their life.

Your tongue should not let harmful food into your body or situations into your life. Instead, it should respond with a 'yuck!' Being a picky eater, in this sense, can be a good thing. Some people aren't picky enough and eat or do all kinds of crazy things, making themselves sick. In other cases, people who are overly picky reject foods, often foods with bitter taste, that could otherwise help them. They don't give themselves enough options and end up eating unhealthy foods. It is the job of the tongue to show you exactly how much pickiness is good for you.

You are what you eat, and that means your tongue is the primary organ that decides the size, shape, and appearance of your body. It is the seat of your health intelligence. In fact, the tongue is called *bodhaka kapha* in Ayurveda which translates to "the bringer of knowledge." You use your tongue to know how your body relates to the material, physical world. That is why taste buds must be treated with utmost respect.

When the primordial Adam and Eve wanted knowledge of the world, they didn't merely look at the tree of knowledge, or touch it - they ate from it. Eating is a profound way to know and commune with the world. By putting the world into your body and digesting it, you incorporate its qualities and characteristics in a way that is unachievable through the other sense organs. The eye and ear perceive from a distance. The nose, closer. Touch, even closer. Taste is the final barrier before the deepest way to 'connect' with the world, which is first and foremost by eating it. The deepest form of connection is communion with God. In the Catholic celebration of the mass, this ultimate communion is accomplished through the very act of tasting and eating God, in the form of the Eucharist.

Somehow, this idea that we acquire knowledge through eating was not lost to the ancient biblical author and it's not lost in Ayurveda. Babies acquire their first knowledge of the world through taste. They explore the world with their mouth. Some babies do this more than others. My youngest daughter seems to put everything in her mouth. She must have a very strong sensory awareness in her tongue. This is true of many people who may not even be aware of it. While some say that seeing is believing, these tongue-oriented people know that tasting is believing, through this most intimate kind of contact. They 'see' the world with their tongue. For others, it's the eyes or perhaps the ears. Maybe your sense of smell is strongest for you. Many of us have a dominant sense organ that helps us explore the world. What sense organ do you 'see' out of?

Strong visions of food come from a strong tongue. In Ayurveda, people with Kapha dosha (the body type in Ayurveda that tends to be overweight) tend to have the strongest tongues. Kapha is one of the three basic body types in Ayurveda, and it is the body type most often associated with weight gain. Kapha people often have very clear vision and clear cravings for food, just like the story, "The Night Before Christmas" when, "visions of sugar plums danced in their head."

My dad has a lot of Kapha. If you mention the word Chinese food when he's hungry, that's it. You can't go anywhere else for dinner because that's what he wants. He won't be satisfied until he's had Chinese food. One time I was cooking for my father, and I told him I was going to make him Ayurvedic pancakes. As soon as I said the word "pancake" he had a specific image of what that was going to taste like. So he didn't like my Ayurvedic pancakes at all, because I put cinnamon and cardamom in them to make them healthier. He couldn't appreciate them because they didn't match his specific vision of what a pancake was going to taste like. So the next time I cooked the very same pancake for him, I didn't call it a pancake. I called it an Ayurvedic griddle cake. He didn't have an association for taste with griddle cake so when he ate the griddle cakes, which was the same recipe, he liked them.

If you're the type of person who sees the world with your tongue, and you have strong visions of food, challenging your food cravings might be a struggle for you, and it requires greater discipline. The next time you have clear cravings or visions for food, take some time to learn from them. Instead of following your impulse and consuming the food object of your desire, explore your vision. You might find meaning in the craving. You might find your craving is emotional. It could even be that the visions of sugar plums dancing in your head are coming from a nostalgic holiday feeling. In that case it is your heart that is hungry, not your stomach. Once you know you have a holiday itch, instead of that deep dish lasagna or your grandma's favorite cookie recipe, you could satisfy that craving with something other than food. Perhaps you might call one of your cousins and talk about old times, satisfying your heart hunger more authentically than with cookies. Maybe you could write your grandmother or sift through some old childhood photos.

Your tongue is an instrument that can lead you into the direction of life and vitality, health and goodness. And it can also lead you astray in the opposite direction. By paying attention to your cravings, food moods, and the taste of what you're eating, you can train your tongue and refine your palate. You can help your body figure out what to each, and navigate difficult food cravings through experience. Over the years, you will enjoy the process of continual discovery, and feel dismayed occasionally by your failures. It is a commitment of a lifetime.

Chapter 5: Experiencing Your Hunger

*

Feast
I drank at every vine.
The last was like the first.
I came upon no wine
So wonderful as thirst.

I gnawed at every root.
I ate of every plant.
I came upon no fruit
So wonderful as want.

Feed the grape and bean
To the vintner and monger:
I will lie down lean
With my thirst and my hunger.

Edna St. Vincent Millay

*

Hunger isn't just a word, it is a feeling. According to the American Heritage Dictionary, hunger is, "...a compelling need or desire to eat food." Your body expresses this desire in many, many ways. Some of the ways your body expresses hunger are simply physical. When you are hungry, you might feel emptiness in the stomach. Or, you might have a hunger pang, which is a physical sensation resulting from contractions of the stomach muscles. Your stomach might growl at you.

But hunger isn't merely a physical sensation, it's also a desire. When you are hungry, your body releases a hormone called ghrelin, also known as "the hunger hormone," which increases your desire to eat. Ghrelin plays a role in reward perception in the same area of the brain that processes sexual desire and addictions. The presence of ghrelin makes eating food feel pleasurable. Ghrelin transforms hunger from a mere physical sensation to a psychological one. To form a healthy relationship with hunger, this psychological component must be examined.

You might start by asking yourself, is my hunger good or bad? The hero or the villain? To many, hunger is suffering and needless deprivation. To others, it is energizing. Good or bad, hunger is evocative, primal, and instinctual. In the book of Genesis, the earth, after its creation, was formless and empty; darkness was over the surface of the deep and the Spirit of God hovered over the waters. Like the abyss of Genesis, hunger feels like emptiness inside, a hollow nothingness. Something is missing and hunger wants to fill it. Yet hunger does not feel simply like emptiness or a lack. It feels like a real presence, and when you feel it, the experience is potent. Hunger can be so raw & powerful it will drive you to eat anything available, just to stave off the ache.

Hunger is something to be explored. Since hunger has so many physical and psychological implications, exploring your hunger is essential to building a healthy relationship with food. Discovering your hunger is a journey filled with many 'Aha' moments of self-discovery. At each step, as you become more aware of and understand your hunger, the easier it will be for you to lose weight. These are important questions which can help you build a healthy relationship with your hunger.

I had a friend from Morocco that could see when a person was hungry, just like you and I can see when someone is cold. I asked how he knew. He said hunger makes your eyes strained & hollow, your eyebrows furrowed. He said a vacant stare signifies your preoccupation with food. The face of chronic hunger is one that is gaunt and impoverished. Hunger reveals the desperation of the body and its utter dependency on food's nourishment. The potency of hunger comes from the frailty and vulnerability of the person.

Hunger is the body's cry for energy. Your body craves energy above all things - the energy to live life. Without this need for energy, hunger would not exist. Therefore hunger has a purpose. It exists to fulfill this need for energy & vitality. If your hunger is true, you should have more energy and vitality after eating. After a meal you should feel motivated and excited to engage in life more fully. That's why, interestingly, the hunger hormone ghrelin is also the hormone responsible for the distribution and rate of use of energy.[4]

Sometimes hunger drives you to eat heavy foods, making you feel tired. People often feel sleepy after eating, instead of energetic. Hunger that compels you to eat heavy food usually isn't hunger for food at all.

---

4 Burger KS & Berner LA, "A functional neuroimaging review of obesity, appetitive hormones and ingestive behavior, "Physiology & Behavior, 136: 121–7.

Instead, it is a hunger for satisfaction and comfort. For many people struggling with weight loss, hunger is no longer a hunger for energy's lightness. Instead, it is a hunger for security and satisfaction. These cravings have nothing to do hunger's real purpose: to give you energy. Instead of craving the lightness and vitality of greens, a person struggling with weight loss may crave the heaviness of eating pizza. Instead of strengthening and nourishing you, these foods make you feel unmotivated.

There are many feelings that pretend to be hungers for food that aren't, which Ayurveda calls 'false hunger.' The hunger for comfort and satisfaction, for instance, feels like hunger for food but it is in reality an emotional hunger. Like false prophets, false hungers masquerade and distort your appetite and food cravings. These false hungers and pathological cravings destroy your energy and vitality, and pervert the original purpose of hunger: to strengthen you and give you life. If you pay close attention to your portions and your hunger, you won't overeat & you won't feel tired.

A potent false hunger is the desire for a full belly. Most likely, you discovered the significance of a full belly as a baby. You discovered that a full belly led to feelings of satisfaction. You enjoyed the energy and fuel that the food gave you. A full belly meant not having to worry about primal needs for a while. It meant safety and comfort. Over the years, a full belly became the solution to many discomforts. Anytime you were feeling empty or lacking, you could fill the emptiness with food. Through this process, feelings of dissatisfaction put on a mask of hunger.

For ancestral humans, the strategy of filling your belly whenever you were tired or depressed was a good one. Scarcity was the norm - there were no ice cream cones in the forest, nor any of the convenient fast food joints that we have nowadays. Fatigue and depression were signs of poverty and exhaustion, signs you needed to eat. Eating when tired and depressed may have been a good strategy, hard-coded in your DNA. In light of modern times, and the abundance of food available in grocery stores, the scales have flipped. In modern times, calories are cheap and only the wealthy can afford to eat light, nutrient rich foods. In modern times, fatigue is not a sign of exhaustion or poverty. Instead, fatigue comes from lack of exercise and poor circulation due to overeating. A candy bar might raise your blood sugar levels for a few minutes so that you feel energized. But as your blood sugar levels and triglycerides rise, your blood becomes thick and hard to circulate, making you feel tired and depressed again. More food brings more fatigue, sluggishness, and depression. Today, if you follow your ancestral impulses to eat when you are tired, you will feed your illness. Unless you are underweight, food will not be an authentic answer to depression or sadness. You can't rewrite your DNA, but you can take the time to notice whether you are really hungry and in need or more food energy, instead of feeding emotional hungers.

Emotional disturbances, sadness, and depression can feel like hunger because they also arise out of desires, or hungers, for comfort. The satisfaction you feel after eating offers temporary respite from your emotions. One of my clients would eat at night whenever she was away from her boyfriend. Their relationship was unstable and her loneliness on these nights only reinforced her feelings of failure and worthlessness. Sometimes the false hunger was manageable - a small bite of chocolate relieved her anxiety. Other times, she sought richer meals including ice cream or cheesecake, which were problematic foods that created congestion and heaviness through the night. It was a vicious cycle she struggled to break.

Pain often masquerades as hunger too. You may have abdominal discomfort, irritation, or inflammation but your brain thinks you're just hungry. Stomach pain feels remarkably similar to a hunger pang, in terms of discomfort. I had a client who ate every time her stomach was hurting. She thought the pain was hunger, but it was really inflammation. When we modified her diet and introduced an herb, her inflammation subsided, the pain was relieved, and her appetite reduced. Even just the realization that it was pain, not hunger, helped curb her appetite. So often, when you become conscious of the false hunger, you automatically start to take the steps you need for a more supportive relationship with food.

Sometimes the false hunger is due to 'taboo temptation.' This is especially true for people fasting from wheat, sugar or other foods. After several days of abstinence you may be pre-occupied by your struggle to resist your cravings, and paradoxically pre-occupied with the forbidden food. If you are fasting from wheat, you may be nearly mesmerized by the sight of a cookie. These feelings of "taboo temptation" can masquerade as a powerful hunger, and one of the main reasons we suggest you avoid crash diets. The temptation to eat forbidden foods are especially difficult to resist in the long term, no matter how sincere your intentions. Inevitably, you will give into temptation occasionally, and create a cycle of feast and famine that is difficult to break, as you waffle between abstinence and binging that ultimately leads you to gain more weight in the end. Instead of abstinence, it is paying attention that is the hallmark of your healthy relationship to emptiness and hunger. That's why crash diets and quick weight loss schemes ultimately fail. In the game of weight loss, the tortoise always beats the hare.

As we mentioned, your body associates many discomforts with hunger. Unless you bring your conscious awareness to them, these discomforts will become impulses to eat. In many ways, instincts are imprecise - they generalize problems and solve them bluntly. You might even hear a voice in your head, "eating felt good last time, let's try that again!" Whether inflammation in the gut or emotional pain - eating can alleviate discomfort temporarily and so, over time, you associate certain discomforts as hunger when they are not truly hunger. Maybe your body simply wants something to make it feel good, even if it doesn't solve the problem. So food becomes a panacea to your brain. Fortunately, you can reduce overeating quickly by noticing the difference between these false hungers and true hungers. It's easy to recognize false hunger once you know how. Just remember: hunger is never painful. It is not an emotion, and it doesn't change with stress. What does hunger feel like then?

In order to know what distinguishes true hunger from other hunger cues, you must first remember the origin and essence of hunger is your body's hunger for energy. Satisfying hunger is not the same as the "comfortable, sedated, full belly" that you may have grown to know and love. True hunger feels more like a craving for refreshment, vitality, and strength. If you are truly hungry, food will not sedate you; it will energize you. Healthy food choices leave you feeling light, energized, and refreshed. You will feel strong, your stamina will be great, and your confidence will not waver. Satisfying true hunger ends in lightness, not heaviness.

True hunger comes from inadequate resources to nourish cells. Any feeling you associate with hunger that does not come from this state of deficiency is not true hunger. An empty stomach, for example, has nothing to do with true hunger when you are otherwise adequately nourished. Many people think hypoglycemia is a sign of true hunger. Hypoglycemia is when your blood sugar levels drop to a point where your body feels alarmed. Although you feel ravenous when hypoglycemic, hypoglycemia is not true hunger either. More often, hypoglycemia is a result of other imbalances, unless it has been at least 6 hours since your last morsel. Whatever you might be feeling in these circumstances, it is not hunger. These false hungers must be discovered and acknowledged if you are ever to discover a healthy relationship with food. Ayurveda says to never eat unless you're truly hungry.

The biological signs of true hunger include a growling stomach, a feeling of lightness, a slight weakness, and coolness in the muscles. If your stomach is not growling, if you feel heavy and lethargic, or if your mind is cloudy and thinking seems arduous, then maybe you aren't hungry. It could be emotional hunger instead. Maybe it's simply dissatisfaction.

True hunger feels like clarity and spaciousness in your mind. The mind wakes up when you are truly hungry and you feel motivated. If your mind feels cloudy and sluggish, you probably aren't hungry. Hunger, by its very nature, is motivating. A lion doesn't hunt on a full belly; he sleeps. True hunger is a drive, a force to be reckoned with. It is not a, "I might as well have another cookie" feeling. Sustained hunger, as experienced on a crash diet or in a prolonged fast, releases endorphins that make you feel high and even powerful, as individuals with anorexia can attest too. Many writers and artists have intentionally chosen a path of poverty because they believed they could not live out their full creative potential on a full stomach.

Hunger is motivating. It gets you up off the couch. Studies show that hunger increases movement in many animals,[5] including humans.[6] Hunger gets you moving. It breaks through obstacles such as sluggishness like no other remedy can. Every time you are hungry, you have to make a choice: should I eat? If you are overweight and tend to be sluggish, we suggest that you harness this spark of energy rather than stuff it down with food. Mild hunger can be a gift, to be admired, celebrated, and enjoyed, like the coming of a sunrise.

In Bangladesh, many people are food insecure. These undernourished souls are experts of hunger. They have a saying, "hunger is the best sauce," which captures the joy of hunger. Water tastes like heaven to the thirsty. Unlike the starvation experienced in extreme poverty, hunger is not a disease. Starvation is when your body cannot get the nutrients it needs, and you start to break down body tissues due to malnourishment. It takes a lot of hunger to get to starvation. Most people can fast for a month or more before they were truly malnourished.

---

5 L. Provencher, & S. E. Riechert, "Short-Term Effects of Hunger Conditioning on Spider Behavior, Predation, and Gain of Weight," *Oikos*, 622: 160-166.
6 G. Wald & B. Jackson, "Activity and Nutritional Deficiency," *Proceedings from the National Academy of Sciences USA*, 30(9): 255–263.

Medically, mild hunger has been shown to increase longevity.

Between healthy hunger and starvation is the feeling of being famished. If you wait too long to eat and skip meals, you may feel like you are starving but in reality you are hypoglycemic. If you are too hungry, or not used to abstaining, your blood sugar levels will crash. The lightness and spaciousness of your mind in this case will change to irritability and anger. While allowing yourself to feel hungry between meals can be healthy and motivating, skipping meals is not advised in Ayurveda. Waiting until the point where you are angry and irritable is unhealthy, unless you are habituated to frequent snacking and need to retrain your body. If you wait until you are famished, you risk becoming indiscriminate about what you eat.

Figuring out how your hunger feels is an exercise that could take several hours, months, or even years. As you delve into your hunger, you will find all kinds of insights into its nature and how it affects your behavior, lifestyle and emotions. What are some of the ways your body tells you it is hungry? How does your body feel when you are hungry? Take a moment to start your exploration of hunger by going through each of these questions, one by one, once a day for a month:

How do I know I'm hungry?
What is the feeling of wanting food?
What does hunger feel like in my gut, heart, and head?
What does hunger feel like on my tongue?
What does hunger feel like in my skin, muscles, and deep down in my bones?
How else is my body telling me it's hungry?

Where is the urge to eat coming from?
Is there a pain somewhere?
Are there emotions behind my hunger?
What are some other things I am feeling besides hunger?

As you delve into these questions, you might start to notice patterns. For instance, you might notice that every time you are hungry, you are also cold. True hunger is cold because your body lowers your metabolism to conserve energy. You'll notice that strong hunger can make you feel irritable, scattered, spacey or have trouble focusing. The more you can notice these sensations and recognize them as hunger (or not), the easier it will be for you to determine when you are truly in need of more food.

Try to get down to the 'poetry' of your urge or impulse to eat. In exploring your relationship to your hunger and body's responses to emptiness, artistic exploration can be invaluable. Art can help you delve into the psychological implications of your hunger. The writer and psychologist Thomas Moore, in his book, *Care of the Soul,* says of poetry "never wants to stop interpreting. It doesn't seek an end to meaning..."[7] We suggest this same relationship with exploring your hunger.

Poetry can help you articulate your feelings of hunger, where they are coming from, and the stories you associate with your hunger. The opportunity for introspection that poetry offers continues to bear fruit as the plot of your personal story unfolds. We suggest you write a whole page of poetry about your hunger, and

---

7 Thomas Moore, *Care of the Soul* (New York: HarperCollins, 1992), 159.

discover the mystery of hunger in your body. Try various art forms. What are the colors of your hunger experiences? How would you sing their song? If your emotions were a dance, how would they move? Would it be fiery like a desert at noon, or a cold, dark, depressing winter storm? Is your anxiety like a dry, cold wind, or is it more like a soggy marsh?

However way you choose to start interpreting your hunger, try not to doubt your feelings and discoveries. You might wonder if the impulses you feel are really there, or if you've imagined them, or if they are too meaningless to be expressed or written down. We suggest, instead of overthinking your experiences and free associations, that you simply enjoy them. Let them run wild, without suppression, and see what comes up. You'll be amazed at what you discover about your hunger.

You may discover you have some resistance to feeling hungry. That you are either afraid of hunger, refuse to let yourself be hungry. Often when I mention the beneficial attributes of hunger and emptiness, clients experience fear even to the point of paranoia. They feel their very survival is threatened. Recently, we hosted a weight loss support group. Halfway through the program, one of our clients posted on Facebook that she had lost her appetite for over a week. Moved by compassion, other members of the group responded to her post. Among the responses we counted 7 suggestions to see a doctor, 5 warnings of dehydration, fears of a parasite or virus, and 1 recommendation to try eating a lollipop. What a great irony in a weight loss workshop that losing one's appetite seems to have raised so much alarm and concern! Personally, I thought it was the success of the program that she lost her appetite. Most likely she was simply metabolizing stored fats and needed less food. We've already mentioned that most individuals, even those of average weight, can survive 3 weeks or more without food. Your body is designed to survive a famine, not that you should put yourself to the test. Within a week this client's appetite returned, and she was several pounds lighter, and feeling energized.

When I ask clients to fast from snacking to experience hunger, many simply protest, "When I'm hungry, I get hypoglycemic. My body can't handle it." Hypoglycemia, when your blood sugar level drops, triggers a state of alarm. Usually, however, hypoglycemia simply means your body isn't used to experiencing hunger. Your body "forgets" it can metabolize fats for energy. Instead of burning these fats, your body wants you to get more energy by eating. Soon you find yourself addicted to snacking - hungry all day long or whenever you use up the sugars floating in your blood. If you follow modern advice to eat small meals frequently, you'll train your body to expect food constantly. The result will be a near frantic dash to the vending machine or box of cookies whenever healthier snacks are unavailable. The pattern of constant 'grazing' is an especially modern one. While your ancestors had to forage for nuts, game, and berries, or dig their food out of the ground, modern food comes in convenient packages. So everyone eats all the time, but this is ultimately very destabilizing for your body and blood sugar levels.

The grazing-all-day culture may cause you to fear hunger, but there is no need to avoid or fear hunger. Buddhist monks eat only one meal a day, proving the body's capacity to maintain stable blood sugar levels over longer periods of fasting. Allow yourself to truly experience emptiness before filling it. Challenge your cravings for heavy meals with a hunger for refreshment and vitality. Mild hunger may have an important lesson to teach you. By embracing emptiness, eating light foods, and fasting between meals you'll soon develop the resilience you need to keep blood sugar levels stable between meals, and hypoglycemia will become like a distant memory. If you are used to grazing, take some time to retrain your body. In fact, you shouldn't try to stop snacking all at once. Just transition gradually.

Many parents also do not allow their children to experience hunger. Frequently these children grow up to be picky eaters. It's easy to be picky when you aren't hungry. When I was a child, my parents wanted us to enjoy Thanksgiving dinner with a big appetite, so they would serve a light lunch to keep us hungry. They knew that 'hunger is best sauce', and wanted me to enjoy the holiday feast on an empty stomach. They knew that food tastes better when you are hungry. Unlike false hunger, true hunger is not picky. Everything tastes delicious to a hungry person. True hunger is also steady; it does not subside. If your child will only eat bread and cheese, chances are she's not that hungry. Allow your child, and yourself, to develop a healthy appetite so that you can discover your true hunger.

Freud defined spoiling a child as not allowing them to work through obstacles on their own. A child who never feels helpless fails to develop true strength. Many individuals still feel this same childlike helplessness into adulthood. They feel under-confident physically and mentally, so they never discover their true limits. But they're not helpless, and neither are you. Your inner child may have a loud voice in your head, undermining your confidence. You may be used to listening to this voice, and believe it is authentically your voice! You may not hear the voice of courage and valor in your chest. If this level of under confidence describes you, hire an uncompromising coach or a motivated friend and start some athletic training. They will help you discover and break through your limits.

As you explore your hunger you can also explore feeling related to hunger, such as lightness, fullness and satisfaction. When you feel light, you feel energetic and vital. Healthy lightness permeates your skin with a cool and airy feeling. Lightness imparts refreshment, as if a fresh breeze were blowing on your forehead. There's a wonderful purity and cleanliness that comes if you allow yourself to be hungry long enough (a feeling that people with eating disorders are addicted to). Next time you feel light, try to feel it all the way down to your bones. If your mind has been cloudy for a long time, lightness feels like freedom and independence. You will feel clear, motivated, and strong.

When was the last time you felt light? It may have been a long time since your last experience of lightness. Unless you have an experience of lightness to remind your body, it will be very difficult to crave light foods. Through a cleanse, a day of light meals, or a trip to the sauna, you can rediscover what feeling light feels like. Once you give yourself an opportunity to feel light again, naturally you start to crave lighter foods again. Journal your experience, so it will be easier to remember later.

After eating, you feel full. When you are full you feel pressure in the stomach, as if the stomach is stretched. As I mentioned earlier, I used to eat until I was stuffed. Consumption satisfied my passion and desire to experience life more fully. Stuffing myself felt great in the moment, but later caused a lot of acidity and irritation in my upper GI. As I learned to eat less, the irritation vanished. Many people, like me, eat so quickly they don't realize they're full until it hurts. To explore fullness, eat slowly and mindfully. As you experience your feelings of fullness, write them down.

Next time you eat, also notice the lull that descends over your mind and senses while eating. Your mind becomes quiet, and the senses, other than taste and smell, are dull. One withdraws inward, engrossed by the blissful experience of eating. Your face relaxes into a blank stare. As your blood sugar levels rise after eating, you can sense the kindness of life inhabiting your body again, replacing the ache of hunger. Satisfaction feels sweet, nurturing and soothing. It is like the gentle pressure of being hugged and contained. This experience is affectionate, like that of a mother's lullaby. In those moments, you become filled with warmth and generosity.

After such a blissful feeling, you want to repeat the experience over and over again and eat too much. When you overeat, the heaviness in your stomach eventually makes you feel sluggish and stuck. Thinking becomes difficult and your brain becomes foggy. You no longer feel the gentle warmth and love of satisfaction, but rather a heavy dullness that is dim and numb. Instead of merely nourishing you, the food has congested you. You feel as if you are living life in a fog, a food coma. You lack motivation to exercise or even to get up off the couch. So, when it comes to satisfying your body, it's important to strike a balance and avoid "too much of a good thing." Just like there is a hormone for hunger (ghrelin), there is a hormone that regulates satisfaction called leptin. Leptin is secreted by fat cells in your body. Leptin naturally regulates your hunger and your weight. Every time you eat a good meal, your leptin levels go up and you feel satisfied. Your body feels safe to let go of any excess weight when leptin levels are normal. But every time you skip a meal when you are hungry or crash diet, your leptin levels go down and you actually become more hungry and less likely to lose weight.[8] Together, ghrelin and leptin function to balance your food consumption. Remember, if you eat slowly enough and when you eat unprocessed foods, these hormones will function properly and keep the balance of your hunger and satisfaction intact automatically.

Notice that fullness and satisfaction are a little different. After so many meals I have been utterly full but still dissatisfied. Isn't that the worst feeling, when you've eaten all the food available until you were stuffed but still feel unsatiated? If you are full but still unsatisfied after a large meal, it normally indicates that some nutrient was missing. It's a good time to check in: what were you truly craving during the meal? What qualities or tastes were missing from the meal - did you want something sour, sweet, light, or dry? Try making a salad, which usually has a variety of nutrients. Or maybe rounding out your meal with a good protein source, like nuts, fish, or chicken.

Sometimes you choose the perfect food, and it hits 'the spot'. When that happens, it's so good. Your food was exactly what you needed and wanted. When food hits the spot, it feels heavenly. You feel satisfaction physically and emotionally. You feel affirmed and on top of the world.

---

8 Jeffrey M. Freedman & Jeffrey L. Halaas. "Leptin & the regulation of body weight in mammals." *Nature,* 395: 763 - 770.

There is a great joy in appropriately satisfying your hunger.

The opposite of satisfaction and fullness is emptiness. What does emptiness feel like? Where is emptiness in your body? These questions are very important because many false hungers derive from pain and emptiness. When your stomach is empty you feel it cramping up. Your stomach growls, then it gets angry and starts to complain. Your solar plexus area may become tight and tense. You feel constriction. If you pay close attention, you can feel your heartbeat in your stomach when it is empty. And consciously or subconsciously, a certain terror arises within you that is primordial, ancient. Where does this terror come from? Emptiness is terrifying because your ancestors endured many famines. Your cells remember the days of these ancient famines and make you feel scared.

The next time you feel the pain of hunger and emptiness, how will you confront it? What is your action plan? Of course, you will feel the impulse to eat. The unhappy urgency you feel makes it difficult to do anything otherwise. However, noticing hunger, lightness, fullness, satisfaction, and emptiness will refine the size your appetite and food cravings. It also gives you perspective on false hungers and cravings, so you can identify hunger as hunger, and emotion as emotion. You can choose how you respond to your impulses once you are aware of them, because you have perspective and therefore freedom.

Most people think the stomach is the hungriest organ, but in actuality, it is not. Have you ever considered how hungry your mind is? Ayurveda believes the mind is the hungriest organ. The mind is hungry for stimulation and experiences. The mind wants to stuff itself full of emotions and productive thoughts. It wants to be rewarded again and again, like a mouse pressing a lever over and over hoping for the candy to roll down the shoot. The mind craves that little shot of dopamine, a temporary sensation of pleasure.

The child on the bike yells, "Look, mom! No hands!" or, "Look at me! I can jump far!" or, "I can do the high dive!" When the child grows up, he boasts, "I can travel the world," or, "I own my own company!" These are all examples of the mind's hunger for glory, its desperation for dignity, and longing to feel special. The mind is also hungry for new experiences. In Ayurveda, the mind is a sense organ, like the tongue. Think of the mind like you think of your hands, your ears and your nose. Your mind enjoys experiencing all the world has to offer it, just like a sense organ. The mind is constantly dissatisfied. It wants to eat spicy food, shop at fancy stores, drink alcohol, flirt with a new acquaintance, and live dangerously, all to distract itself from dissatisfaction. It uses the other five senses to touch the world, and feels happy when it discovers something new and useful.

For many, the greatest emptiness, threat to survival, and obstacle to weight loss is loneliness. A study published in the Archives of Internal Medicine found a correlation between being alone and worsened health outcomes.[9] Loneliness triggers such a great sense of shame and failure that people sometimes eat just to feel better about themselves. Loneliness may be so acutely painful that it is very often the tipping point from overweight to obesity. Of course, being alone is different

---

9 Carla M. Perissinotto, Irena Stijacic Cenzer, & Kenneth E. Covinsky, "Loneliness in Older Persons: A Predictor of Functional Decline & Death," *Arch Intern Med.* 2012, 172(14): 1078-1084.

from experiencing loneliness. Loneliness is when you are alone but long to be with someone. You feel it right in the center of your chest, as if an elephant is sitting on you. Loneliness is a sinking feeling. Your chest and shoulders slump. It feels damp and cold, so you want to crawl under the covers and sleep. Loneliness makes a person feel undesirable and flawed. They feel worthless and ashamed of themselves. So they eat food to reassure themselves. Tasty food reassures them they have a good life.

Since humans are social beings, loneliness is a natural feeling. You can be together with many people and still feel loneliness, because the mind is never satisfied with the love and affection it receives. This is why you must train yourself and your mind to be grateful. What each of us is going through is so similar. That should be reassuring - to remember we're here together. We all pray each and every day, each in our own way, for relief. Reconnecting with God can help to restore your hope, which is a very beautiful thing. Hope, like love, is a verb. You have to practice it. Hope is what allows us to wake each day with new eyes and new experiences, believing wholeheartedly that you can find deeper connection even though you feel alone in the moment.

The next time you feel emotionally empty, how will you choose to respond? How long can you tolerate emptiness? How deep can you go into your emptiness? Are you afraid of the emptiness and its void? A poem on hunger may only fill a page, but the depths of emptiness could fill a whole book. The mind abhors emptiness. To confront the mind, ask yourself these questions: how willing are you to do nothing? How willing are you to have an empty life? How willing are you to feel separated from that heavenly satisfaction? Of fullness?

Emptiness and dissatisfaction are altogether frightening and many times we eat because emptiness feels like failure. We believe that our very survival depends on fullness and satisfaction. Emptiness is a place that most would prefer to avoid, because we associate it with suffering. We want to avoid that pain because pain, like emptiness, is often feared. But if you listen to your pain, you'll learn from it. My herbal teacher, the late Frank Cook, used to say, "Feeling pain is feeling life." He always said that pain is the sign of your will to live. Are you willing to feel the pain and emptiness of being alive? New research is showing that people who are obese are also more sensitive to pain. They have a lower pain tolerance. Obese people may feel more urgency to fill the void of emptiness right away.

But emptiness is not the abyss of nothingness. Fullness is dull; it is already completed. Emptiness is the beginning. It offers refreshing possibilities. It is awake, alive and expecting. We may fear emptiness because in emptiness there is always uncertainty. A baby deer wobbles on her legs as she tries to walk; infants fall hundreds upon hundreds of times before walking on their own. Emptiness can feel scary because it is a little unsteady. But if you can sit with the uncertainness and unsteadiness, knowing that in the end it's all going to be "ok," then you free from its power.

Pope John Paul II talks about man's insatiable desire to participate in the blessing of life, to have all the abundance of nature. It is helpful to remember that this condition of desire is a shared experience that we all have. It is a condition of being human. Your sense of deprivation and that deep desire to participate in the beauty and wonder of creation is a sacred craving shared by all. The desire for life is truly beautiful. It is the truest of all hungers. Man is hungry to know the Creator of life, so he can have life and escape emptiness. Yet, the shortcuts - whether avoidance, denial, or doubt - appear like so many tempting false hungers before us.

The question remains, how much of life are you willing to experience without sedating yourself? Are you willing to love the pain of your desire without suppressing it? Are you willing to be empty physically, but awake and aware of the pain of life? You can find peace in emptiness if you choose see it with new eyes. Emptiness, just like hunger, is not a disease. Instead, it reveals who you are, and where your passions lie. In Matthew 6:21 Christ exclaims, "For where your treasure is, there your heart will be also." When you know your emptiness, you know your desire and treasure. You know your heart. It may be that emptiness is your only access to the secrets of your heart. If you suppress this voice, and your hunger, you will never know yourself. If emptiness is truly the voice of your soul, suppressing it amounts to rejection of your deepest desires. Instead of suppressing or escaping it, show your emptiness some compassion. Cultivate a new relationship with emptiness, one that is kind, and nurturing. Emptiness may be impulsive at times. Be kind to it anyway. It is your inner child, after all. By cultivating awareness of its tantrums, you can care for it, as you would a baby.

Tomorrow, perhaps for the first time, try experiencing emptiness. When you get hungry, try waiting a full hour to eat. Set your watch to beep every ten minutes and write down your thoughts and feelings. Bring plenty of patience with you on this exploration. Then enjoy your food. You've earned it.

*

Unconditional

Willing to experience aloneness,
I discover connection everywhere;
Turning to face my fear,
I meet the warrior who lives within;
Opening to my loss,
I gain the embrace of the universe;
Surrendering into emptiness,
I find fullness without end.
Each condition I flee from pursues me,
Each condition I welcome transforms me
And becomes itself transformed
Into its radiant jewel-like essence.
I bow to the one who has made it so,
Who has crafted this Master Game.
To play it is purest delight;
To honor its form--true devotion.

Jennifer Welwood

Chapter 6: The Nature of Desire

*

Experiencing emptiness and becoming OK with your hunger is an important part of any weight loss journey. Alongside emotional emptiness and physical hunger are your internal impulses and base drives. Awareness of these impulses brings insights into your behavior patterns and the strength to change them. In fact, without becoming aware of your impulses and desires, it may become very difficult to lose weight and, more importantly, to grow as a person and reach your full potential. But, what do we even mean by an impulse? An impulse is an urge to do something; it's the force behind the craving to grab a cupcake. The force is raw, willful and strong. When you are aware of your impulses, you have an opportunity to examine them, and have the freedom to choose whether and how to satisfy them. When you are not aware of your impulses, you lose the freedom to make a choice.

Perhaps your impulses are conditioned after many years of practice, like desiring to eat doughnuts after church or to drink a cup of coffee in the morning. It may be an urge to have a glass of wine when you get off work or enjoy dessert after dinner. Whatever the object of your desire, an urge or impulse is that little voice in your head that says, "I want THAT...and I want it now." Discovering your internal impulses, interpreting them, and dealing with them helps you establish healthy behavior patterns with food. Hunger, the desire to eat, is a formidable impulse. As you study your impulses you will penetrate down to the very roots of your actions & behaviors, giving you yet another edge on liberating yourself from unhealthy false hungers.

The theme of how to deal with urges, impulses and desires is not unique to Ayurveda, but is central to many religious traditions. Liberation from desire is the major theme of Buddhism, for example. The major difference is that Ayurveda treats your impulses as a physical phenomenon, instead of merely psychological or spiritual. Rather than pondering the ethics of desire as religions do, Ayurveda examines the physical experience of it. "What does desire feel like?" Ayurveda tries to make sense of your desire physically and trace it back to its biological roots: is there a biological imperative behind your cravings - a nutritional deficiency, an impaired organ, or stressed tissue?

To be clear, there is nothing wrong with desire. Being in touch with your impulses means you are in touch with your instincts. Ayurveda believes that a person's thoughts, emotions, and physical ailments are all related, and that your desire may be expressing a legitimate biological need. This connection between you and your body helps you understand your biological needs and therefore how to nurture yourself. Still, instincts and impulses can get distorted and lead to illness and weight gain. Distorted instincts can be very difficult to resist. An examination of your inner drives and motivations can shed some light on your eating habits, and help resolve some distortions in your hunger.

Let's examine an example of an urge. Imagine it's a cold, crisp November afternoon and you are walking home from a hard day at work. You stumble across the local bakery and there, in the windowsill, is an absolutely decadent four-layer chocolate cake. The texture appears rich, soft, and creamy. Instantly, you are swept away by desire to eat it - a fantasy of eating delicious chocolate cake swirls around your mind which is so evocative you can almost taste it already. You imagine biting, tasting, and swallowing the luscious cake. If you're like most people, your urge to eat the chocolate cake catches you off guard like a doe caught in headlights. Everything else fades into the background except for you and the irresistible object of your desire. You might feel like you are somehow entranced, or even trapped by the thought of pleasure. You may become fixated on getting exactly what you want.

Advertisers know that people are mesmerized by desire. A TV ad presents you with video clips of fresh, hot pizza that it is utterly seductive, creating an urge in your mind to eat the pizza. Lust may seem like a strong word to describe your urge to eat the chocolate cake or pizza, as lust often has a sexual connotation. Yet, food cravings are by nature pleasurable and can seem irresistible, much like sexual desires. Like sexual lust, desire to eat a chocolate cake can have a forceful quality to it that seems difficult to resist. There is a primitive nature and raw urgency behind food cravings.

The next time you notice strong desire to indulge in food, take it as an opportunity to also recognize the sensations of desire. Desire increases and then dissipates again, like a slow wave. When your desire is strong, you might feel overwhelmed. In that moment your senses become fully engaged. Your mouth starts to water and salivate. Desire is warm. The next time you feel desire, take a moment to notice these sensations in your body.

Deep down, the power of desire is alarming. In the moment, desire feels difficult to control. Because of its potency, resistance to desire may seem futile. You may feel compelled to devour the chocolate cake. Urges, by nature, are very demanding, domineering and unreasonable. No one likes to feel out of control, and often in the face of desire for food, you can feel overwhelmed and maybe even afraid of the base instincts driving desire.

All humans have them, yet urges seems primitive, pre-human, and uncivilized. The urge to eat is a primal and instinctual drive that we all have. They are the proverbial "bull in a china shop" - savage, impulsive, and brash. Urges operate on an instinctual, animal level, what author Sandra Maitri in *The Enneagram of Passions & Virtues* calls the "primary subjective reality, your basic needs & wants existing prior to any interaction with the world." When the urge has you in its grip, you are mostly wild animal and infant. You feel all sense of propriety is lost. The urge itself operates at the border between biological need and psychological want. It cuts through all the fluff and gets down to what is basic & elemental. It lacks refinement or subtlety. Maitri points out that, in the childlike simplicity of an urge, there is nothing beyond avoiding pain & seeking pleasure. The world is divided into sources of gratification and obstacles to gratification.

In this state, your libido may become belligerent with any obstacle to gratification, including obstacles such as other people. No matter what obstacle is in your way, you will find a way around it in order to get the chocolate cake. Your desire overlooks any inhibitions you might have, forcing you to do things you would not normally do, like eating a whole chocolate cake or pizza. Desire is a welcome and seductive distraction from life and its many struggles. Once I gave a client an herb called Gymnema, which temporarily destroys your ability to taste sweets. The next day she came home stressed out from work, and wanted a brownie to calm down. Because of the herb, she couldn't taste the sweetness of the brownie, and became angry and upset. My client had to deal with her stress from work rather than suppressing her feelings with a brownie.

You can distract yourself with food and find a moment of "bliss" when you eat rich, indulgent foods like cake. This simplicity is adaptive in some ways - they "get the job done." Urges are direct, bold and courageous. Yet desire ignores reality and your better judgment. You might quickly forget about the consequences when entranced by a decadent treat. Often, you can convince yourself that the indulgence is ok - "just this once," you might say. Urges have a certain rebelliousness to them - the rules don't apply to urges. You may also derive some security knowing you can have what you want any time you want.

Some people fear deprivation- and the suffering they will have to endure if food is not readily available. Food cravings frequently mask survival anxieties. I remember as a young boy I would always cut the line at a buffet because I was afraid all the 'goodies' would get eaten up before my turn. Children will cry for sugar as if their life depends on it. Survival anxieties may creep up as you pack for a vacation. "What if I haven't packed enough food for the trip? What will I eat for lunch?"

Some people make frequent trips to the grocery every time they run out of an ingredient, just to feel secure they can get what they want. Are you a person who naturally hoards foods, especially sweets and treats? Challenging these survival anxieties helps soften the tension around them.

Perhaps your desire comes from feeling bored or under stimulated. When you are dissatisfied or bored, pleasure brings relief. Desire is often rooted in some other dissatisfaction with your life. We all want to believe we are capable of stronger feelings and greater emotional responses. We all want to feel alive. You may feel as if your cravings reconnect you to your more sensual side. Sometimes cravings for food are a reaction to feeling dry. You may fear that if you don't indulge your desires, you will miss out on the pleasures of life, that your sensuality might dry up, and that you will become numb and robotic. You may fear that if you don't follow your temptations, you are being stingy with yourself. Food is one of life's greatest and most sensual pleasures. You may feel that you have to indulge because there are no other possibilities or means to live life sensually and fully. Trying to fix your dryness can lead you to become "promiscuous" with food, indulging in rich, heavy foods despite lack of hunger. Try to notice when your desire is merely a reaction to feeling this kind of emptiness.

Strangely, some of my clients desire indulgent foods more when they lose their appetite. When they lose their appetite they become confused, unsure of what to eat, what to avoid, and how to experience pleasure without food. When that happens, instead of following their body's natural cue for abstinence, they seek out food that's ever more decadent, food that promises not to disappoint their need to feel & experience. They eat more chocolate cake trying to get that feeling of satisfaction they crave. People are often alarmed when food loses its appeal. Everything makes them feel dissatisfied. They feel they have nothing else to fall back on when they feel bored. But certain times of year, it is natural to lose your appetite. So often loss of appetite is simply a sign that your body is metabolizing fats and detoxing. Your appetite and joy of eating will surely return when this process is complete; you just have to trust and put faith in your appetite. Try not to fear dieting; please and enjoyment will return soon. Addressing and relaxing into this fear of loss helps to abate unruly fits for food pleasure, and helps you discover healthy ways of fulfilling pleasure that support your body.

Sometimes urges and food cravings are biological or hormonal. A woman may feel the urge to eat during certain parts of her cycle, especially when ovulating or during a hot flash. Some people crave sweets and heavy foods at night after trying to eat light foods all day while on a diet. Whatever your cravings are, you must find its source, whether physical, mental, spiritual, survival, or hormonal. Once you've found its root, you can unearth its mystery and heal its power. Ayurveda offers a number of great ways to cool your passions. To help you sober up so you can think again, try splashing some cold water on your face. Or, try herbs with bitter taste like neem. Bitter herbs are an effective way to quell excessive desire in the moment.

Before you can get perspective on the desire you are feeling, first you have to wake up from its trance, much in the same way a pinch can help a person wake up from a dream. This is more difficult than it sounds. When desire has you in a trance, it's hard to think of anything else. Once you wake up and find some perspective, try to express and write down your experience so you can name it. Pay particular attention to any physical sensations, emotions, and beliefs that well up. Throughout your examination, notice each of the qualities (called gunas in Ayurveda) of your cravings. Are they heavy, light, sharp, dull, hot, cold, oily, or dry? Do you notice any patterns like a frequent craving for something heavy and cold? Light and sharp? Oily and dull? This exercise provides provide important information about your physical state, which an Ayurvedic practitioner can help you with. You may also start to notice how your cravings correlate to imbalances you are having.

When these sensations come up, enter into the emotions of your desire fully but without indulging it. You will notice that your desire is like a little child crying and pleading for lollipop. Ask yourself, "How would I deal with a little child throwing a tantrum?" If you give a kid a lollipop every time he cries, the child will learn that it can get what it wants by crying. You teach the child that crying is an effective strategy for getting what he wants, therefore training your child to cry. But if you can wait through the discharge of pent up energy, letting the child cry without giving it the lollipop, you may discover other ways to reassure the child with your love, or why the child is really upset. Perhaps the child is hungry, or tired.

The same is true not only with a child and a lollipop, but also with your mind and what it wants. When you show your desire some patience and willingness to experience temporary deprivation, you find the motivation and willingness to discover what is truly behind your desire or dissatisfaction. Once you are able to feel your emotions, they naturally subside. By being soft and gentle with your emotions, you put yourself back in the driver's seat, instead of letting your emotions run wild. You regain control of yourself, your feelings, and ultimately your life just by bringing awareness to the emotions you are having.

As you start to examine desire, painful shame may well up inside. If you haven't been able to control your habits, the loss of self-control can trigger feelings of failure and disappointment. You may feel embarrassed by the social taboos preventing you from acting on your urges and impulses. You might want to hide the evidence of the chocolate cake or candy wrappers because exposing your lack of control makes you feel vulnerable. No one wants to examine desire, or even talk about it. However, by delving into these feelings, you will find ample opportunity to learn about yourself and the roots of your desire to eat. That will give you the insight you need to overcome the feelings of disappointment and failure.

When it seems difficult to shake the thought that the chocolate cake will bring the perfect satisfaction you crave, remember that desire is 90% fantasy. Desire works by harnessing the power of your imagination. The excitement of desire disturbs your ability to think rationally. Though still a fantasy, desire feels substantial and real. Sometimes, after satisfying your desire, you feel frustrated or incomplete. Consumption may not measure up to your imagination. The real cake seems disappointing when compared to the fantasy one. Often, the fantasy itself is the most enjoyable aspect of desire. If you eat the chocolate cake, you'll merely suppress the joy of your fantasy. Desire itself is pleasurable, and should be thoroughly enjoyed before satisfying it. After you've examined your desire and sat with it, you can make a decision about whether to fulfill it or not. Like water breaking through the dam, the inevitable bite of chocolate cake discharges the fullness of wanting, a catharsis as the urge is liberated. Once satisfied, the energy of desire dissipates, and life returns to a quieter, uninspired state.

You may be aware of bad habits, but you don't know where they came from, why they are there, or how to control them. You may feel that your body is out of control or that it has betrayed you for wanting to eat unhealthy foods. The mysterious origin of your desire leaves you feeling victimized by your bad habits. You may believe you are unhealthy due to bad luck or fate. To penetrate these mysteries it is natural to ask, "Where does desire come from?" Ayurveda suggests that the desire or impulse to eat unhealthy food is not simply the whim or fate of your body, but actually has origins which are explainable and fixable.

One such explanation of desire is that it is triggered by your body trying to relieve tension. When you feel the strain of a long day at work, your body triggers desire for relief which can manifest as a food craving. Desire, which may seem whimsical, often stems from such underlying physical discomfort. In this context, desire's purpose is to trigger a search for relief - a search for medicine. To demystify desire, you have to find the underlying discomfort. Once you find the underlying discomfort, you can also find a healthy way to provide relief.

For example, you might crave chocolate because it seems to offer relief both physically and emotionally from a long day's work. In examining your desire for chocolate, try to find this discomfort, which may feel like tension

111

somewhere in your body. In that area you will feel tightness, pressure or even a dull ache. You may notice the tension in your body makes you feel mentally squeezed, and like you have no time or space left to operate in the situation. The discomfort you feel triggers your search for an immediate solution, which manifests as forceful desire often projected on food. This tension is the essential ingredient giving desire its urgency and power.

The tension may arise in various parts of your body but particularly in your head, chest, & gut. Can you feel any tension in your head, chest or gut right now? Your urge may also come from joint pain flaring up, a stomach ulcer, or some other painful sensation. Take a moment to make a list of all discomforts in your body, and notice how they make you feel emotionally. Tension in your heart area makes you feel like your chest is being squeezed. Tension in your stomach can make you feel nausea or butterflies. Tension in your head makes you feel distracted and stressed. Your body will want relief from these discomforts, and trigger food cravings as an antidote. The power of your cravings can mask these hidden physical roots of your impulses to eat. Your mind wants to eat the chocolate cake instead of facing the real problem - the seething cauldron of emotions and tensions beneath.

Similarly, beliefs that rationalize eating the chocolate cake - "I deserve a little dessert" or "a few bites won't hurt" - also well up from physical discomfort. These rationalizations seem like objective truth, but in reality many of the beliefs we take for granted are feelings triggered by underlying physical and emotional states.

Nobody wants to admit their beliefs are emotional because they seem so real in the moment.

Meanwhile, how do you deal with that sense of fullness, excitement, and adventure that desire seems to promise? Until you experience the relationship between your emotions, your beliefs and your physical body, you will continue to feel that the source of your food cravings is a mystery. You will feel frustrated by your food cravings. You will feel exhausted by the stress of your emotions. And your beliefs will lead to unsupportive behaviors. Unexamined impulses drive you to do things that are healthy. When your urges come from subconscious feelings they are also distracting. Until you understand and address the roots of your habits mentally, physically, and spiritually, the habit will be hard to break. Remember to look for underlying tension whenever you have a food craving, so that you can provide a real solution to your discomfort instead of a food based Band-Aid.

In my clinic, I help clients find the physical tension, emotions, and beliefs that are at the root of their maladaptive relationship to food. I help them discover opportunities for self-examination when desire for food is triggered. They learn to face the physical and emotional beliefs they are feeling - so they can identify their impulses and behavior patterns. For example, a client reported that around 3pm every day she thought about eating sweets or snacks from the vending machine. The craving felt so strong and overwhelming that she often ate the food despite knowing that it will not make her feel good. After a few weeks of working with her, we discovered that around 3pm she also had a pain in her abdomen that she never realized before. By helping her notice the abdominal pain, she was able to realize how her food craving was an attempt to soothe the pain. Recognition of the pain helped her resolve the craving.

Another client of mine would often get into arguments with his wife. He was unaware he had a dull ache beneath his right rib cage, in the liver area of his body. Once we found the ache, he started to correlate the ache with feeling emotionally disturbed and irritable. He told his wife about it so she could remind him. Now when he feels irritable, she reminds him to poke his liver. He follows some gentle exercises to flush his liver. Once you realize how your food cravings are triggered, you can address the real issue also, and overcome unhealthy cravings. For example, a 15 minute walk midday helps relax your body at work, so you never feel the strain, its emotional consequences, or the desire to fix it with food later in the day.

Next time you have an unbearable food craving, start the discovery process of finding tension, discomfort, and sensations in your body. Sit down, close your eyes, and take a deep breath. A breath is a great way to release the grip of desire. This breath creates a gap between desire and action. Even a single breath can create a moment of patience. Loosen up your neck and shoulders. Scan your body from head to toe, paying particular attention to the head, chest, and gut. Then scan your crown, forehead, throat, heart, solar plexus, lower belly, and pelvic floor. Finally, notice your muscles and skin. Check both the back and front of your body. Do you sense any discomfort, pain, or tension somewhere? Try giving the tense area a nice self-massage. This can release the tension and will ease the intensity of the craving.

We have all heard of the "count to ten" principle. A breath and counting to ten can help you recognize the desire in the mind without acting. It creates the space to find any physical tension in your body, to notice the emotions you are feeling, and examine the beliefs you use to rationalize your actions. Soon, you'll feel the desire begin to soften and subside. As you gain perspective through this process, you will also grow in your strength and stability. You become more able to artfully handle life's many challenges.

When you stay in the gap between desire and action, you start to free yourself from your own prison. Desire is not a state of free will. Immediate gratification is often thought of as a type of freedom, so to speak: I wanted what I wanted, and I went and got it." You feel unfettered by the rules of the world. Unfortunately, the truth is that you may be more enslaved by desire than you think. True liberation is the freedom to make great choices for yourself, free from compulsive thoughts and desires.

It is easy to become a slave to desire, a slave to what you crave. You might know that something is not good for you, and will lead to your unhappiness but you do it anyway. Because desire is so inviting, you don't acknowledge the deceit and suffering until too late. If you had true free will, you would feel free to choose the path to your ultimate happiness, and avoid paths that lead to suffering. When you are not able to choose that, there is a loss of free will, even if you are following your desires without restriction. In the context of food, true liberation means the ability to choose healthy, delicious, satisfying food that is life-giving.

Desire makes you feel alive and abundant because it seems sensual. Yet, at the same time, haphazardly satisfying every desire you have for food desensitizes you. The more you indulge the senses, especially taste, the duller they become. Not too long ago we were teaching Ayurveda on a cruise ship. If you've been on a cruise, you probably know already that temptation is everywhere. On this cruise we ordered a slice of warm, gooey chocolate cake every evening for 5 days. The first day the cake was absolutely amazing. By the 5th day, the cake made us feel sick. We took one bite and couldn't eat any more. I felt sad that I had somehow destroyed, by overindulgence, my appreciation for this culinary delight. If you mindlessly eat a cookie every day with your lunch or dinner, the cookie will start to lose its appeal over time. It becomes less and less special and exciting to you; it is no longer a treat, but merely a habit. You lose the rich pleasure of the cookie, and may start feeling like you need two cookies in order to get the same pleasure that the single cookie formerly had. Indulging desire for food in this way is a never ending cycle, because desire is never satisfied. You will merely crave more and more stimulating experiences to get the same pleasure you once enjoyed from just one.

When a special treat no longer seems special to you, it is a sure sign of overindulgence. Instead, reignite your passion for food by waiting. Abstinence for several days can help you restore your sense of delight. Saying grace before eating can also help restore specialness, meaning, and a sense of the sacred to the treats you eat. Don't just mouth the words - or mindlessly chew your food. Instead experience the sacredness of every morsel you eat. Let appreciation be the root of your rich, sensual life. The chocolate cake is something beautiful, sacred, and precious. With appreciation you will find more meaning in your pleasurable experiences. Develop a daily practice to re-awaken spiritual connection and meaning beyond consumption. Food isn't mere fodder to fill an empty stomach, it is cuisine to be admired and appreciated.

How will you know whether desire is healthy or pathological? Is it the healthy, cellular hunger that is felt deep down in your bones? Or is it a quick fix? You can, and should, indulge some of your food cravings because your body might be communicating with you real nutritional needs. But which ones? The skill to discern the difference between healthy food cravings and pathological desire may take a lifetime to master. Nobody knows the precise formula to liberate you from your desires. If you've struggled with food cravings, you are not alone. Try to appreciate how difficult it is for anyone to overcome compulsive behaviors and forgive yourself. It takes hard work to resist the desperation of desire.

An anonymous quote states that "the difference between seduction and true love is that seduction leads you astray, and true love brings you back home." What is that home? It's your true calling. We all want to fulfill our highest goals, and live the life of our dreams. Like true hunger, this kind of desire is sacred. Other desires are merely seductive, and prevent you from reaching your full potential. Sometimes, it seems one must wait forever for fulfillment. This longing for fulfillment is excruciatingly painful, like pining for true love. So often, we don't even know what will fulfill us, or where to start looking for true love.

Gratification for this or that is a seductive alternative when true fulfillment seems unattainable or too far in the future. It seems easier to gratify the senses with food, out of frustration and impatience, so you might as well eat a piece of cake. Desire that comes from frustration and impatience with life is lack of purpose in motion. You can't rush your journey through life. Settling for second best comes from fear that you will never have the answers, that you will never find fulfillment. On some level, you know that in every indulgence, you are giving up on something better. There are no shortcuts to the discovery of your true purpose and mission in life. A certain guilt may arise afterwards if you are satisfying desire that isn't authentic.

Next time you have a food craving, take a moment to reflect: will gratification truly fulfill you? To overcome the fantasy of desire, try to hear God's calling in your life. The founder of Saks Fifth Avenue David Campbell writes, "Discipline is remembering what you want." By examining your desire, it slowly unfolds into a real, substantial passion for what is true. Your will start to recognize your true purpose in life. By avoiding shortcuts, you harness the powerful energy of desire and redirect it to the object of your true love. You avoid distractions that sap your energy and refocus on realizing your true goals. Similarly, examining your food cravings slowly unfold into passionate awareness of true hunger. Take a moment to experience your desire for food. Will the chocolate cake truly fulfill you? If yes, you have found your passion for chocolate cake. If no, your desire is incomplete. Wait patiently until you find a more vital option. When your love is true, it brings delight to your very soul.

Chapter 7: Emotional Eating

*

Using food to cope with mental anxiety, fear, anger, depression or other emotions is known as emotional eating. Many people eat emotionally because their emotions are difficult to cope with, and food seems like a quick and easy way to avoid the discomfort. You may be having difficulties in your relationship, at your job, or coping with loss. The emotions you feel may be powerful; and when you have them, they are stressful. Even mild emotions can be disruptive. When you feel fatigue dealing with the stresses of life, or feel anxious from a recent quarrel, you may be tempted to use food to calm down or "get rid" of the emotion. But when you eat food for emotional reasons instead of nutrition, food becomes medicine to provide comfort, or to relieve insecurity, rather than to nourish your health and well-being. Like the desert mirage, food appears to offer relief - but it ultimately is a false promise and in fact, emotional eating can make your emotions worse rather than better.

Let us explain how this works. I once had a client who drank beer whenever she was with friends to help her relax and have a good time. She was drinking the beer for emotional comfort, not because her body needed it. After the beer, she'd want to smoke a cigarette. And after she had a cigarette, she would begin to feel agitated and have intense emotions. By the next day, she would be eating ice cream, cookies, or chocolate to calm the agitation. This client thought she had a food addiction, a smoking addiction, and an alcohol addiction. But after several sessions we realized she just had social anxiety when spending time with friends. Once we addressed the social anxiety, she overcame these addictions. The story of my client illustrates how social eating or drinking can affect your normal diet and routine, and also trigger uncomfortable emotions.

Have you ever heard the popular children's story *The Woman Who Swallowed a Fly*? In that story, one thing leads to another - the dog eats the cat that eats the spider that *"wiggles and tickled inside her. She swallowed the spider to catch the fly, perhaps she'll die."* The emotional eating in the fable snowballs to catastrophic proportions, much like the frequent insanity of how emotions unfold. We've all been there, and have experienced the same downward spiral after a party or a night out with friends, even if it did not model this client's experiences.

Emotional eating takes many forms. Stress, strain, and fatigue are one of the major causes of weight gain that we see every day in our clinic. Our overweight clients report again and again that their work schedules are so demanding they don't have any time to eat healthy foods, or to digest their meals. In addition to being overworked, our overweight clients also report too much stress. They are stressed out and eating to cope with stress, which is a type of emotional eating. They don't have enough time or energy to cook a nice meal, sit down, and enjoy.

Once, I had a client who would binge after a long day at work. I asked her to journal her emotions right before binging. The next time we met she brought her journal, and we discussed how she was feeling. We discovered that her stress & emotions were due to eye strain. After a long day staring at the computer, her eye muscles were strained and exhausted. The strain made her whole body tense. She was using food to calm herself down. With some simple afternoon eye exercises to relax and de-stress her eye muscles, and adding a fifteen minute break in her afternoon routine, she stopped binging. Ayurveda reminds us it's important not to overlook the physical body when finding solutions to emotional instability. When your body is strained beyond capacity, you feel strangely disconnected from other people and even your own feelings. You feel as if food is the only way to settle down and feel like a human being again.

In addition to stress, you may eat to distract yourself from physical pain or discomfort. Whether you eat or drink to relax around friends, like my client, after a long day at work, or even for fun when you are simply bored, anytime you eat without real hunger, it is a kind of emotional eating. Eating food for entertainment, like popcorn at a movie or due to a social obligation such as hors d'oeuvres with friends, is also a form of emotional eating. When going through an emotional or strenuous time, a person may notice themselves eating more in general - they may start getting seconds on meals more frequently or snacking more regularly. This is also a form of emotional eating, even though it may seem more "under-the-radar."

To be clear, it's OK to eat for emotional reasons occasionally. A conscious choice to eat for entertainment or emotional comfort in certain situations is normal. Food can soothe you when your stomach is tightened into knots. It can settle your nervous system when you feel vulnerable, fearful, or unsettled. Food is a way to bring you into your body and out of your head - replacing anxious, scattered, restless thinking with a physical sensation - so that you can feel your body again. Food can be very reassuring. That's a good thing, in fact, especially for Vata-predominant people who tend to live in their head and get lost in inspirational thoughts and ideas. A warm bowl of mashed potatoes with ghee may be just the thing they need to come back to earth. It is a convincing way to tell your body, "I'm safe. Everything's OK." And after a little bit of food, everything does feel OK temporarily. Your belly is heavy and full. Your mind gets a temporary diversion. When something unexpected happens and you are not sure how to react, eating can provide a temporary fix. Sometimes it's the only thing you know how to do.

When your emotions are triggered, you may feel like you need to get rid of your feelings right away, and re-establish your composure. Maybe you messed up at work and you are disappointed in yourself. Perhaps you are going through a big break up, or are suffering the loss of a loved one. Maybe you are simply anxious or you feel a vague sense of dissatisfaction with your life. If your aversion to these painful emotions is strong, these feelings will put you in an intense state of need - you will have an emotional hunger for relief. Just like food hunger, you may feel driven & compelled to satisfy this inner urge to run away and avoid the emotion by any means available, including food. However, since the cause is emotions rather than lack of food, eating doesn't help. Emotional eating, consciously or unconsciously, is eating to fulfill what we called a "false hunger." When you are emotionally eating, you are not truly hungry for food. The true hunger, emotionally, is abiding tranquility. The fulfillment you seek is not a satisfied belly, but a satisfied mind. Emotional and spiritual hunger ultimately cannot be filled with food. Any temporary fix to these festering hungers only prolongs your suffering.

Furthermore using food as a way to escape what you don't want to feel can become an addictive habit. If you emotionally eat too often, it can create health problems. Your body may not be able to process the food well, leading to digestive or other health problems. Emotional eating can cause unintended weight gain, high cholesterol, and high blood pressure. It can make you feel tired and depressed.

Are you the type of person that uses food to shut your mind off? Fortunately there are healthier ways to achieve this. One method is self-massage. While sitting, you can try to rub the tops of your legs and you may find it very soothing. You may find that it brings awareness back into your physical sensations. Sometimes I rub my fingers through my hair or give myself a gentle scalp massage, which can be very soothing. Any time you rub your skin, it moves blood around, increases your circulation and cleanses your lymphatic system. This relieves not only stress but helps you to feel refreshed. You can give yourself a little backrub, or you can rub your tummy or just hold your belly and feel the warmth of your hand...that works really well in the winter on cold and frigid days. There are lots of options to get out of your head and into your body. Sitting out on the porch, taking your shoes off and walking through the grass, or holding a loved one's hand - those are all ways to get out of your head. You can also engage in some gentle exercise, perhaps through a restorative yoga class. All of these are ways of getting back into your body and quieting the anxiety, even if for only a short period of time.

Once you feel settled, however, it is still vitally important to re-examine your emotions. As much as suppressing your emotions prevents you from knowing your patterns and dealing with your own struggles and insecurities, all the emotional unrest and the eating that follows will continue to keep reoccurring. Life is difficult, and stuff is always coming up. Taking a moment to feel your feelings is therefore worth the investment, even during the busiest days or during the most stressful times.

When things are going well, dealing with emotions seems easy. But when things start to unravel or fall apart, you may fall back into old habits. During these difficult moments, following through is difficult to accomplish. Specific triggers and emotions can cause you to eat in a frenzied, sad, or otherwise emotional state. The next time you are triggered and feel like you are losing your grip, create some space with a single breath. That simple pause will create an opportunity for perspective.

Ayurvedic offers great into how your emotions and your body are connected. If you struggle with emotions, or are emotionally sensitive and don't know why, Ayurveda can provide answers. Sometimes, the emotion you are wrestling with comes from an imbalance in your body, not your psychology. Bodily imbalances make your emotions more intense. Imagine having a splitting headache. Your daughter runs into the room, screaming and crying. Would you be able to handle that situation more gracefully if you didn't have a headache? Or, imagine that you have a runny nose and have been stuffed up and bed-ridden for days. You are totally miserable. That night happens to be the night your you have a disagreement with someone, and you completely lose your cool. Wouldn't it have been easier to manage that situation if you weren't also battling a cold? You are more equipped mentally, physically, and spiritually to deal with emotions, pain, and conflict when your body is in a state of balance. When we become sick or imbalanced, maintaining poise becomes a little bit more dicey and difficult.

Unfortunately, many of the foods people eat when emotional are foods that lead to imbalance, and make their emotions worse. Though it might seem hard to believe, food dramatically alters your personality, how you think and behave. Some foods like wheat or dairy congest your blood flow and can make you feel heavy, lethargic, depressed, tired, or even panicky. Other foods, like celery, make you feel energetic, optimistic, and light - perhaps even ungrounded if taken in excess. Some foods, like pumpkin or sweet potato, make you feel calm and peaceful. Some fiery foods like chili peppers, tomatoes, coffee, or chocolate may aggravate you and lead to anger, irritability, or frustration. Each food has a personality, and by eating that food, you perhaps unknowingly affect your personality.

My dad loves to go out for Barbeque when he visits me here in Asheville, North Carolina. We had gone out to his favorite barbeque restaurant called 12 Bones. I had the pork barbeque and he had the beef brisket. 12 Bones is famous for its barbecue sauces and we enjoyed every mouthful. Everything was great - but about 15 minutes after eating we got into a fight. We were talking about politics, and probably we were both right but couldn't see each other's point of view. We got on each other's nerves. Whatever I had to say seemed so important at the moment that I couldn't just say, "Yes, OK" and move on. And he couldn't either.

Halfway through the confrontation I realized how emotional I was. My emotions seemed out of proportion to the conversation we were having. It seems there was something compelling me to fight. The fact is I just couldn't let it go, even though my relationship with my father is more important than politics. There was something preventing me from keeping calm. Then I remembered we had both just eaten a large plate of red meat with spicy barbecue sauce. Meat, especially red meat, can make a person stubborn and unyielding. Red meat is so hearty that it builds overconfidence and pride. Its iron builds the blood and creates great enthusiasm and zeal for one's beliefs. If a person eats red meat every day, they're going to be a beefy, hearty person. To boot, fiery barbecue sauces irritate your intestines and can make you irritable.

In that moment I realized that it was really the effects of my pork barbecue fighting with his beef brisket. It's so tempting to think that it was my dad's fault that caused the altercation. In truth, probably I could have been more forgiving of our difference in opinion had I not been fired but by spicy BBQ. People always the choice of how to respond, but sometimes, because of intense emotions, forgiveness is difficult to achieve. Difficult situations provoke you to feel certain emotions. However righteous your emotions may be, Ayurveda believes your ability to respond appropriately is a measure of both your maturity and state of balance. In the situation with my father, the food we ate undermined my ability to respond maturely. This is because the food you eat, and the imbalances in your body, can make it difficult to get the right perspective.

Ayurveda believes the intensity of one's reactions is determined by imbalances of blood chemistry, often due to food. Passion is in the blood, so they say. Although there are times when intense emotional responses are correct, it is the exception not the rule. Careful consideration of your inner state of balance, self-control, and perspective on the situation at hand can help you freely choose how to respond. Even recognizing that I was fighting not because of the topic but because of the food that I just had helped me to let go of some of my emotions and stop the debate. This recognizing is important. In the recognition everything begins to change.

Here's another example of how this works: one hot summer day, I remember having a spicy chocolate brownie with my lunch. About two hours later, I noticed myself getting very tense and frustrated at everything and everyone around me. I could feel anger welling up within me for some unknown reason. I was wondering why I was getting so upset, and then I realized that both chocolate and cayenne pepper are very fiery ingredients. They are a little bit irritating. In the hot Southern summer, in the middle of the day, it was anything but medicinal for my body. Take a moment to consider what you've eaten in the last few hours. Can you own physical and emotional changes from these foods? Your answers will change based on the food, the season and your unique constitution.

Often, maintaining a balanced mind and body is as simple as balancing your blood chemistry. Eating healthy foods can help you maintain stable blood sugar, protein and triglyceride levels. Staying hydrated, maintaining good bowel health, and abstaining for caffeine and alcohol are also good ways of keeping your blood clean and balanced. For those who wish to take balancing their body to the next level, follow the right Ayurvedic diet for your body type. Your emotions will become mellower as your blood reaches a more balanced, healthy state.

Ayurveda describes the emotional relationship between food and your mind through the concept of sattva, rajas, and tamas. Sattvic foods are those which quiet your mind and create clarity. They are things like organic, fresh fruits and vegetables, and greens. Sattvic foods help a person feel more spiritual. Performing sattvic actions like volunteering, taking care of loved ones, praying, saying the rosary, meditation, practicing yoga, listening to calm serene music, and spending time in nature are also ways of bringing about a calm, balanced emotional state. Rajasic food triggers movement and action, yet also chaos and disarray. Rajasic foods are things like red meat, chocolate, coffee, garlic, and chili peppers. They activate your mind and can make you hyperactive. Even though some rajas are good, too much rajasic food makes people more emotionally volatile and scattered. They may make a person want to dominate the people around them. Rajasic actions are things like working in a high stress business, doing intense workout regimes, or behaving in a controlling or domineering way.

Tamasic foods lead to lethargy, congestion, depression, sadness. These foods are generally heavy and sleepy, like pasta, bread, cheese, dairy and fried foods. Tamasic foods make you feel stagnant and stuck. Tamasic foods are what people normally turn to when they emotionally eat

Remember that each taste affects your mood in a unique way. If the blood is sour, it can make you feel envious or jealous. If the blood is salty, it can make you feel sturdy and bold. If you eat too much food that is spicy and hot, it can make you feel passionate, courageous, or even irritable. If you eat bitter foods, you might feel more light, clear, and independent. If you eat too much bitter you will feel withdrawn and bitter at the world, almost like nothing in the world is right. The lines between emotions, blood chemistry, and food are blurry.

It is ironic that people who eat emotionally know, more than anyone else, that food has the power to change their emotions. It seems that emotional eating is proof that food has the power to change the way you feel. It's important to recognize, if you eat emotionally, that you already believe food can make you feel better. You may even have believed in food *so* much that it got you into a bit of trouble. Nevertheless, the good news is that Ayurveda agrees with you. Food does have the power to change you. Food does have the power to alter your personality - and you can harness that belief and use it for your own transformation. Ayurveda is the art of choosing food according to the experiences and feelings you want to have - to improve physical, emotional, and spiritual balance. Ayurveda offers a vast comprehensive means to explore the way in which food affects you emotionally. Through Ayurvedic understanding, you can begin to explore the relationship between personality and food, and then use food to mellow emotions which are too intense.

The fact of the matter is that food, after digestion, becomes blood. Then the blood feeds your whole body, and all of your organs. The blood feeds your nerves and brain, so small changes in blood chemistry have a powerful effect on your mood. It happens that nerve tissue is one of the more sensitive tissues in the body. So any time blood chemistry changes, your whole nervous system changes. As much as food becomes blood, and feeds your organs, it changes who you are and how you feel. You are what you eat; your brain, your heart and your whole nervous system and all of your emotions are affected by the food that you have eaten.

If your blood is heavy and watery from water retention, you may notice you feel sad and depressed more often. If you eat foods that depress your metabolism and make you feel cold, you'll notice that you also feel fearful, insecure, and anxious. If you eat foods with caffeine that stimulate the release of stress hormones you'll soon notice that you have a hyperactive personality, are more easily stimulated, awake and mobile, or even stressed, agitated and jittery. If your blood is sweet from overeating nourishing foods like candied sweet potatoes or pumpkin pie, you may notice you are predisposed to feel affectionate and compassionate towards others.

My mother is wonderfully empathetic; it is one of her best qualities. Years ago, when she was walking on the beach with my nephew, she came across a bird who had broken its wing and could no longer fly. My mother became distraught and overcome with pity for the bird and could think of nothing else except getting the bird help as soon as possible. As her quest to help the bird began to fill the evening hours, my nephew became very hungry. As the hours passed, he got hungrier and hungrier and began crying until my mother finally relinquished and found food for him. If your blood is sweet, you'll find it very easy to be compassionate, and can even get overly compassionate sometimes. You may even be distracted from taking care of other things at hand because you are too compassionate. That sweetness of blood is a wonderful quality as it makes us loving, compassionate and affectionate people, but overly sweet blood can lead to undue attachment as well. We need to maintain a balance of sweetness otherwise it could lead to emotional eating.

Food not only has the power to change your blood chemistry and the power to change your mood, it also has the power to change your whole personality. Start to notice how your personality changes a few minutes or even a few hours after eating. Set a stopwatch for 15 minutes, then for an hour, and two hours after eating. Pause at those times to see how you feel. If you tend to eat the same food day after day, your food-induced mood becomes a way of life that changes how you think. Over time, the food choices you make shift your beliefs.

I grew up in an Italian-American home. We had tomatoes or tomato sauce every day. A tomato every day changes you over time. Tomatoes are acidic; they're sour. They change the bile flow and liver chemistry, which in turn alters your blood chemistry, making blood more alkaline. It affects metabolism. Tomatoes make a person more fiery, romantic and passionate. Even if it is very subtle, if you eat a tomato almost every day for a year, you'll probably notice over time that your moods will change. Your thoughts will change. And the change in your thoughts will cause a change in your habits, and some of your beliefs as well.

Similarly, if you drink coffee everyday then it will cause a change in your personality - making your tense and hyperactive. If you drink coffee every day, you'll start to believe life should be lived in the fast lane. Over time, you will begin to believe, "I need energy. I need to be stimulated. I need to move. I need to move fast. I need to be mobile. I need to be upwardly mobile, progressing, climbing." That's what I call a belief system! A change in your beliefs may also cause a change in your friends and social circles as you gravitate towards people with similar beliefs. If you drink coffee every day, eventually you might find yourself in a social group that has those same beliefs you do, or who buy into what coffee offers. People who drink alcohol frequently are much more likely to have friends who also drink alcohol than to have friends that abstain. I've even had clients who believe their entire marriage would fall apart without their morning coffee ritual. But none of this reflects your authentic personality. It is a false identity. You would have to introduce yourself as, "Hi. I'm Jane plus coffee," instead of just Jane.

We all know that substance abuse changes your mood, how you think, and your beliefs. But it is true in regards to certain foods and food addictions as well - there's a whole belief system and personality surrounding them that sometimes you need distance or separation from. When people are recovering from alcohol addiction - they can't hang around in bars with the people they used to hang around with. The more powerful the substance, the stronger the personality shift and the stronger the addiction.

So how is food affecting your personality? If you drink coffee every day, it's going to be really hard for you to know the personality effects of coffee until you abstain for a week or perhaps even a month. If you abstain for a whole week and then you add coffee back in, you are going to know what a personality possession by coffee feels like. Or if you don't eat sugar for a whole week, then you reach for sugar - you are going to know what possession by sugar feels like. Similarly with bread, cheese, potatoes, pasta and other comfort foods. You have to abstain to know how it is affecting you. This week, try abstaining from one food you believe affects you emotionally. Then you can decide whether you like the change. See what life is like without this favorite food. An elimination diet helps you return to your original, natural and wholesome state, so that you can be yourself again. Then, journal your experience and see what you discover.

If you aren't yet convinced that emotions and the body are related, think of The Incredible Hulk, the comic book hero who came to life on 80's daytime television and more recently in a feature film. When his anger is aroused and he metamorphizes into the hulking green giant, he makes a fist, clenches his arm muscles, tightens his stomach, and brings all that energy right into the solar plexus of his body. He expresses anger in his pursed lips, a furrowed brow, and the tightness of the pectoral muscles of his chest. By looking at his stance, body language, and facial expression, you already know how he's feeling. When angry, most people feel tension in one or more of those muscles. It is as if the body holds anger in these areas.

Before modern medicine, common folk knew a lot about how emotions were stored in their body. Colloquial sayings still reflect those observations: a person might be "a pain in the neck," have "a lot of gall", or be "weak-kneed". A person might lack a backbone, have a thick skull, or maybe thick skin. You might recall feeling your "stomach tied in knots", or having a "strong gut feeling", or being "stabbed in the back" by a friend who betrayed you. When something inspires you, it 'takes your breath away'. Maybe you feel 'choked up' by something sad. These sayings suggest, albeit implicitly, the strong connection between emotions and your body.

Ayurveda claims that every emotion - whether anger, bitterness, loneliness, or betrayal - is held somewhere in your muscles and organs. The shoulders and neck store stress as constriction. And the sternum holds sadness when it droops. You may experience sadness in your heart, or anxiety as butterflies in your belly. Emotions live in your body just as they live in your mind.

If a certain emotion is making you eat too much, try to figure out how you are expressing this emotion physically. Whether it is anger causing tension and tightness, or sadness causing droopiness and flaccidity, releasing your muscles and adjusting your posture helps you overcome the emotions. If the Hulk could simply relax his chest and biceps, he would feel more relaxed. Military generals know that standing erect, shoulders back will increase the confidence of the soldier. Studies in psychology show that people who stand upright or stand in a stereotypically "powerful" position report feeling more confident and bolder than people who slouch and cross their legs.[10] This suggests that changes in

10 Amy Cuddy, Caroline A. Wilmuth, & Dana R. Carneyk, "The Benefit of Power Posing Before a High-Stakes Social Evaluation," *Harvard Business School Working Paper*, No. 13- 027, September 2012.

musculoskeletal alignment can change how you feel. Ayurveda studies this science of the emotional-body connection very carefully. You can too.

Take a moment to recall a recent emotion you've had. Now ask yourself, the following questions:

1) What is the emotion that you feel?
2) How did you know you were feeling that emotion?
3) Where do you feel it in your body?
4) Are you able to release tension, or lift the sagging muscle in this area?
5) How do you feel after this change?

At first, the emotion might seem difficult to locate in your body. Often, the tension is more subtle than it appears in the Hulk. You might feel dull pain, a sharp pain, a gnawing or scraping sensation, heat or coldness, pressure, emptiness, or your pulse throbbing in a certain area. It can be helpful to remember that every emotion you have shows up in at least three places: your heart, head, and gut. You may feel it in other places as well, but you should always attempt to feel it in each of these three areas. The Incredible Hulk probably feels it in his biceps, but you may feel it in your throat - like a lump in your throat. Maybe you feel it in your thigh, your shoulder, or your back.

The second question above might sound peculiar. You can tell someone, "I was really mad today." But how did you know you were angry? How would you describe what being angry feels like? You may say, "I don't know. I was just angry." But in fact, you were probably feeling about 10 different things which your body instantly and intuitively recognized as signs of anger. Next time your anger is triggered, try to put together a list of these different sensations. If you know the 10 things that are happening in your body, you become more conscious of your feelings and emotions. Building awareness of these signs can help you unwind some of the unconscious holding patterns that cause your distressing emotional states to persist longer than necessary.

Like the Hulk, until you can notice and relax the tension in your chest, biceps, and furrowed brow, you may have difficulty letting go of your anger. If you are physically stuck, you may be emotionally stuck as well. As you identify the physical sensations - or felt sense - of the emotion, you can start to uncover the mysterious mind-body connection that masks your emotional eating patterns. Journaling is a very helpful tool as you begin to recognize muscle holding patterns you experience repeatedly. Through proper alignment of your musculoskeletal system, you can start to unwind the powerful grip an emotion has on you.

Remember, the Ayurvedic approach to emotions is body-centric. Through massage and other techniques, you can find relief from incessant anxieties. Through diet you can balance the passions in your blood. By understanding how your body and your emotions are related, Ayurveda helps you feel calm in the midst of a crisis.

Chapter 8: Food Addiction

*

Some foods have the same effect on the brain as alcohol, nicotine, heroin and cocaine. They stimulate the reward centers of your brain. These foods, when consumed repeatedly, can create an emotional and physical addiction. They give you a 'hit' of pleasure just like a person who takes a hard drug feels good temporarily after taking the drug. Food addiction is the most extreme form of false hunger. It is a real and present problem in our society and has the potential to create real problems in your life. Unlike other addictions, such as alcohol, food addiction is particularly challenging. A person can live without drugs and alcohol but a person cannot live without food. Everyone has to eat. Abstinence is not an option as with alcohol.

Most people have an addictive tendency in one or more areas of their life. Addiction takes many forms. People can be addicted to alcohol, social media, work, or illegal drugs. It could be shopping, or an addiction to beauty care. Some people may even be addicted to inspiration, exercise, or an adrenaline rush. Regardless of the form, addiction makes a person feel out of control. You may feel like a failure. You may say to yourself, "I'm bad. I can never get it right." You may feel like you have let yourself or someone else down. Then guilt and shame well up. All forms of addictive overeating usually involve some feelings of guilt and shame afterwards.

The foods that cause food addiction come in many flavors and varieties but we'll explore the most noxious ingredients and addictive additives. For one, processed food is especially addictive. Processed food generally includes anything that comes in a box, anything that you can't find growing on a tree or that was once alive in its current form. Some examples of highly processed food include crackers, candy bars, chips, and ice-cream but there are many others. Most of the foods in the center of the grocery store are highly processed.

Some of the main addictive ingredients found abundantly in processed foods are sugar, salt, and fat. Sugar, salt, and fat have been called the Unholy-Trinity for their addictive tendencies. It is the precise combination of these three ingredients that make a processed food especially compelling. Food scientists have a term, called a bliss point, for when these foods are the right ratio to each other. Too much sugar makes a product too sweet. Not enough sugar is equally unappealing. The bliss point is the amount of sugar, or any ingredient that optimizes palatability - giving you the greatest pleasure. Michael Moss, author of *Salt, Sugar, Fat,* explains that sugar is essentially a legalized narcotic. Studies have shown that mice will work as hard for corn oil mixed with sugar as they will for cocaine. Sugar, Moss claims, acts as a stimulant. It is the "methamphetamine of processed food ingredients". Fat is the opiate, "a smooth operator whose effects are less obvious, but no less powerful." Salt is stimulating and also has addictive tendencies. Your taste buds adjust to salt so you need to keep eating more to get the same effect.

Sugar and all high glycemic index foods release dopamine, serotonin, and endorphins in your brain - natural opiates that make you feel good. These chemicals are the same chemicals released by cocaine and other drugs. They temporarily relieve discomfort, anxiety, and depression. They can give you either renewed energy, physical relaxation or a sense of well-being, depending upon the food. But for anyone who has ever eaten too much sugar, you already know too much sugar creates a transient "sugar high" followed by a subsequent dip in energy making you want to more sugar and starting a vicious cycle.

Even though people don't think of bread as sugary, a slice of white bread has the same effect as 5 tsps. sugar. Two slices is equivalent to a can of soda. Dairy products, especially ice cream and cheese, also contain lots of sugar. Sugar, grains and dairy foods dramatically raise blood sugar. An inevitable crash follows. The blood sugar roller coaster you experience after eating these foods can make you emotionally unstable, and also leads to a physical dependency.

In addition to impacting blood sugar, some foods can have morphine-like effects on the brain. For example, dairy products contain casomorphins. Wheat and other gluten grains contain gluteomorphins. Both of these compounds are opiate-producing, and create withdrawal symptoms when you stop eating them, according to Dr. Aristo Vojdani.

Many substances override your body's natural appetite suppressant mechanisms. A classic example is high fructose corn syrup, a common sweetener in many processed foods. So, if a person has a coke made with high fructose corn syrup with their meal, they may never feel full and will thus keep eating and eating and eating but never feel satisfied. Have you ever had a soda from another country? What you'll notice is that sodas in other countries are made from pure cane sugar, not high fructose corn syrup, and are much more satisfying and nourishing. They fill you up, unlike American sodas which turn you into a bottomless pit. It has actually been directly linked to the obesity epidemic because it fools the consumer into thinking they are still hungry when they have actually consumed more than enough calories to feel satisfied. If a person struggles with soda, switching to pure cane sugar soda can be a good place to start in breaking the addiction. Health food stores often have sodas made with cane sugar and organic ingredients, so those can be a better option too.

Poor quality fats, such as trans fats, can also cause addiction. Most companies know that trans fats are bad for your heart, but still occasionally add trans fats to foods because they "improve" the taste and addictiveness of the food. They are often added to desserts like pastries to make them more "flakey" and tasty. Another cause of food addiction and skewed appetite is pharmaceuticals. Certain drugs can lead to specific, bizarre food cravings while others may increase your appetite yet slow your metabolism, leading to weight gain and a poor relationship with food.

Some foods are addictive because of the way they stimulate your senses. Your feelings of satisfaction depend upon how your sense organs are stimulated, a term called sensory specific satiety (SSS). This means the preparation and presentation of food can be just as addictive as the ingredients. The idea is to create appeal on multiple sensory levels. When food is appealing enough to your sense organs, you might end up eating a whole bag of chips, even if you are already full. Even when you are satiated, flavor enhancers like MSG and artificial food coloring can entice you to eat more food, often beyond your capacity. Artificial food coloring creates visual appeal, like brightly colored candies or cupcakes. High-end restaurants often create beautiful, artistic plate arrangements that please the eye and entice the customer. Foods such as ketchup have many stimulating tastes like saltiness, spiciness and sourness. The food industry also adds carbonation to beverages to make them more stimulating. Sometimes they will make foods so gooey, like chocolate chip cookies, that they become very difficult to say Altogether, the feeling and textures of these foods create an irresistible allure.

Some foods are addictive because of novelties in every bite. For example, cookie dough ice-cream creates intrigue with every bite. You never know when you are going to get a satisfying chunk of cookie dough. Foods like Doritos avoid a specific, single flavor so that you don't get tired of eating them, as you would with too many bananas or a more mono-taste ingredient. By delighting your palate in a dynamic way, these foods become very hard to put down and keep you coming back for more in the future.

Softer foods that require less chewing trick your brain into eating more. When you can eat food very quickly, your brain thinks you haven't eaten very much. That is why the food processing industry designs food with just enough chew – but not too much. In effect, the food processing industry has reduced the average number of chews from 25 times to 10 times. To make foods softer, the food processing industries adds enough fat so that they literally melt in your mouth. Scientist Steven Witherly described this phenomenon with the term "vanishing caloric density." He notes how, "If something melts down quickly, your brain thinks that there are no calories in it . . . you can just keep eating it forever." Examples of these melt in your mouth foods include Cheetos. Cheetos, he notes, seems to melt away after you eat it. You just keep popping one after the other in your mouth. Ice cream is another example. Think of a soft piece of Wonder bread, a hunk of cotton candy, or a smooth piece of chocolate - it literally dissolves in your mouth and, therefore, creates some lingering dissatisfaction when it disappears just a little too quickly. These foods keep you begging for more.

Other techniques that the food industry uses to get us addicted to their products include making foods crunchy. Crunchy foods delight many of us. This craving for crunchiness is actually medicinal. Natural crunchy foods are normally high in fiber and are cleansing diuretics, like celery, cucumbers, and even popcorn. Nuts are crunchy. Even though they aren't cleansing they are a healthy whole food. Crunchiness in natural foods sometimes signifies freshness, which is pleasing. A craving or addiction to crunch may indicate that you need more cleansing or that you are retaining too much water. It could mean you need stimulation, as chewing especially on crunchy things wakes up the mind. The food industry creates artificial "crunch" in foods like potato chips, kettle corn, and crackers. However, these artificially crunchy foods do not offer the same benefits as crunchy foods in nature, which confuses your body.

Many factors increase your chances of becoming addicted to food. Genetics play a role, as well as family history of addiction. Was your house stocked with healthy foods as a kid? Did your parents reward you with food? Environment and culture plays a role. Do you have access to healthy food in your neighborhood? Do you feel social pressure to eat unhealthy foods? You should also consider the way your parents framed your relationship with your body and food when you were younger. Did your parents make disparaging comments about your weight when you were young? Did they try to limit the amount of food you were allowed to have, or make comments when you were eating? Did you have to finish everything on your plate? This kind of "food police" treatment during childhood can set a person up for erratic, addictive, or emotional food behaviors later in life.

It seems that even something like an allergy can cause us to strongly crave certain foods. Even food allergies can cause food addiction. Often people are addicted to the very food they are allergic to. A client had an allergy to beef. After several years of abstaining from beef, the thought of a hamburger seemed heavenly to him. Another client had a mild citrus allergy, and yet craves citrus often. If she does have an orange or grapefruit, she will immediately crave another one even though it always causes GI distress and other imbalances. Some people with wheat allergies crave gluten.

Addictive food cravings often beget other addictive tendencies. A common addiction we see in our clinic is the classic wine and coffee spiral: you feel tired in the morning so you have a cup (or multiple cups) of coffee, but the coffee revs up your adrenal glands and so you get stressed out throughout the day, feeling tense and anxious. By the end of the day, you are so out of your wits that you need a glass of wine to wind back down and relax. But wine creates fatigue and more exhaustion, so you wake up the next day needing a cup of coffee to get going. And the cycle continues. It's easy to get lost in these kinds of spirals.

Alcohol and the caffeine in coffee are both drugs, but food can create a similar spiral. Eating sugar, wheat, or heavy comfort foods may provide some satisfaction and contentment initially but afterwards these foods congest your body & depress your circulation, leading to depression and a sense of sadness and tiredness. Then you end up eating those comfort foods again to overcome the emotions of depression, or eating other food to get more energy. But then the food actually doesn't give energy but just weighs you down more, compounding the feelings you were fighting to begin with. So, you eat more but nothing seems to help you get back on track or put the spring in your step.

People often become addicted to foods when their body isn't functioning very well. Ayurveda asserts that all addictions can come from weak function of an organ. It could be a disorder like diabetes, insulin resistance, or a hypothyroid that triggers you to overeat certain foods. Maybe you overeat because your kidney is not functioning well, or your lungs are a little bit weak. Your heart may not be functioning well. Parasites, especially candida, make you more emotional and hungry all the time. You could simply be tired from a long day's work. When a part of your body isn't functioning well, that puts stress and strain on your body, creating discomfort and anxiety. Even your ability to process emotions can be weak. You may feel easily overwhelmed or stressed.

Unfortunately, when an organ is weak or tired, your body naturally craves something to stimulate it, to compensate for that organ's weakness. A person with a weak liver might become addicted to alcohol, because alcohol stimulates the liver. People with weak adrenals crave coffee. A person with weak lungs craves cigarettes. And a person with a low thyroid or weak adrenals craves sugar. Unfortunately, chronic alcohol consumption makes the liver weaker, caffeine makes them more exhausted, cigarettes cause lung cancer, and sugar depresses your metabolism. These things "stimulate" the function of the organ which is necessary if it is underperforming, but they are also toxic to the organ and hurt it. So, you need a better solution.

To remedy the addiction physically, you have to identify what part of your metabolism and organ metabolism is poor so that you can restore strength to that part of the body. If your adrenals are weak, it probably means you are under too much stress. You can restore strength to your kidneys by resting them. If your thyroid is too low, it can mean you aren't getting enough oxygen. Breathing exercises and other mild exercises can reduce blood stagnation and congestion, helping to balance your thyroid. By supporting these organs you can reduce your sugar and caffeine cravings.

Some people are addicted to food due to an oral fixation. Freud talked about the oral stage of development in infants – when the child is obsessed with oral stimulation. During this stage the infant is satisfied by nursing at the breast. If the nursing child is not allowed to breastfeed, the infant can get stuck in the oral stage of development. And in some cases, the child may seek oral stimulation into their adult life. In other cases, the child may have been overprotected and given the breast too much to calm them down, or to put them to sleep. In the first case, the child may have anxiety about being nurtured by others and being dependent upon others. In the second case the child is over dependent upon others and doesn't want to ever experience any kind of suffering.

If you know you have an oral fixation, then you have an opportunity to discover other, non-food based, ways to self-soothe. Can you think of some other things you can do for comfort besides that oral stimulation? It could be a comforter - a warm fluffy blanket you can snuggle at night. It could be a warm cup of tea, or snuggling someone you love. Performing a nightly *abhyanga* or full body oil massage before a hot bath can help soothe your nerves and anxieties. Perhaps it is kissing your beloved. Some of those still involve an oral fixation, but it doesn't involve food. Or, an affirmation like "I am safe. God will protect me." Use the same method of reassuring yourself every time, so you can develop a new habit.

Ayurveda offers the following advice for medically recognized signs of addiction including obsession, compulsion, denial, increased tolerance, and withdrawal symptoms. According to the Oxford English Dictionary, an obsession is "an idea or thought that continually preoccupies or intrudes on a person's mind." Obsession is one of the important signs that a person is addicted. A person obsessed with food is constantly thinking, planning and worrying about food. They may visit the grocery store several times a day, or panic when food isn't available. They love to talk about food more than any other topic. But just thinking about food or looking at pictures of food could lead to an increase in cravings and appetite.[11]

For many people preoccupied with food, any stress or anxiety makes them feel suddenly hungry. If you're like that, recognizing you are just nervous instead of hungry will be a challenge. One way to tell the difference is by looking for signs of hunger in your blood, instead of your belly. Notice whether you feel weak and a bit lightheaded from low blood sugar levels. That might be a more authentic hunger measuring stick.

If you still find yourself thinking, obsessing, or dreaming about food, it is important to first consider whether you are receiving adequate food and a well-balanced diet, well-distributed throughout the day. Do you purposefully skip meals or suppress your hunger? Are you overly restrictive with your foods, eating only small portions and avoiding rich, sweet, or nourishing foods out of fear? Sometimes, an obsession with food comes from eating too little calories in the last few meals. Other reasons could be a history of yo-yo dieting, eating nutrient deficient foods, financial insecurity, and even starvation might leave you feeling scared or uneasy about food availability. This survival anxiety becomes a false hunger to eat. The food insecurity that results can have powerful psychological effects that lead you to become obsessed with food. Since obsession is often due to erratic feeding behavior, obsession with food is a Vata body type disorder.

---

11 P. Schüssler, M. Kluge, et al. "Ghrelin levels increase after pictures showing food," *Obesity (Silver Spring)*, 2012 Jun; 20(6):1212-7.

A good example might be someone from the Depression era; the persistent, suppressed hunger from a poverty-stricken childhood often leads to a fixation on food, a "finish your plate" mentality, stinginess, and a general unease when food is unavailable during adulthood. The residual fear of this childhood impoverishment lingers even after finances and food intake has stabilized, leading to a tendency to hoard food, overstock the fridge unnecessarily, or a general uneasiness without food.

Hoarding, constant planning of meals, and preoccupation with food can be traced back to our utter dependence on food for survival. Some of my clients came from families that didn't have enough money to buy food, or were neglected as a child. But for most of us reading this book, famine is not our current reality, which is why anxiety based hunger is often false. Yet many people, at various points in our lives, have experienced strong feelings of hunger evocative of food deprivation whether or not these feelings reflected true risk of starvation. Whether due to your own temperament, actual poverty or neglect you may have developed a mentality of food scarcity. One way or another, food scarcity can linger on as an obsession with food in your adult life, creating a false hunger for food.

Ayurvedically speaking, a strong routine is one of the best ways to reduce general food anxiety. I remember when I was growing up, I would get very hungry. I was one of those kids who got hungry ON TIME (and was ready for food). But I grew up in family that had a very erratic schedule for various reasons. My parents are wonderful people, and adventurous but not very schedule oriented. I remember being ravenous as a kid and experiencing that feeling of "I really need to eat." Even if you know you won't starve mentally, your body may still react strongly. An erratic schedule may trigger stress hormones that lead to general anxiety in your life, even if you are otherwise well fed and mentally stable. A good routine makes you feel more confident. A routine reassures your body that it will be adequately fed, which at the same time allows your body to experience hunger between meals. In Ayurveda we say that a good routine is the foundation of a well-lived life. A good routine allows you to plan your meals and plan your life, bring health, wealth and happiness. The foundation of a good routine includes both a meal routine and a bedtime routine. A mealtime routine means scheduling your meals at the same time each day, with minimal snacking in between. A bedtime routine means that you get in and out of bed the same time each day, regardless of whether or not you are sleeping. With these two pillars of a good routine in place, you'll notice your food anxiety will gradually subside. Routine is a very advanced study on Ayurveda, far beyond these pillars, which is part of every practitioner's lifestyle training. The better your routine, the more stability and balance you will create in your life.

Working through body image issues can also help free you from an obsession with food and also from yo-yo dieting, so that you don't swing back and forth from crash diets to binge eating. A person with body image issues or yo-yo dieter needs reassurance that their body is safe, secure, beautiful, and loved just the way that it is, or else they could continue to struggle. Learning to love your body, attending body image and empowerment workshops, and spending time each day speaking kindly to your body can be very healing. Coming to peace with food is also crucial. Even after losing weight, a person pre-occupied with food is still at risk for gaining weight again. Until their obsession with food is truly healed, their relationship with food will be hard to manage.

Many people, instead of dealing with their anxieties, develop compulsive habits that provide temporary relief. Compulsive behavior is defined as doing something repetitively even though it doesn't give you the reward you seek. These compulsive habits feel good, but distract you from dealing with the underlying anxiety directly. It is one of the signs of addiction. One of my favorite quotes, famous from Alcoholics Anonymous, states, "Insanity is doing the same thing over and over again, expecting a different result." In compulsive overeating, food is usually a coping mechanism for some kind of stress. You might be coping with past traumas, financial stress, or any other kind of stress. Eating provides temporary relief, but it doesn't fix the underlying emotions. To boot, compulsive overeating can lead to excessive weight gain.

Many of my clients with compulsive overeating talk about their eating habits as if somebody else was doing it. They feel like something takes possession of their body, compels them to eat, and then they wake up 20 minutes later having eaten a whole bowl of food. They feel as if their mind has gone blank, and they have no control over portions. It is as if they have lost awareness; lost consciousness. Actually, it's an altered state of consciousness where eating becomes automatic and one loses the free will to make a choice about whether or not to eat. It is a kind of trance-like, zombie state, exactly like the trance of desire. Many people know this happens to them, but they may not know why it happens or what to do about it. It may just seem like they're a victim to whatever force has taken over their body. Due to the forceful nature of compulsive behavior, compulsion is a Pitta body type disorder.

Trances are more common than you think. They happen whenever emotional triggers put you into a reactive state. When I ran my first company, I remember receiving an angry call from our investors one day. It was my first company, and I had made a mistake. They were right to be angry. But I was so upset I ate a whole burrito just to calm myself down. I couldn't even think straight because I felt so deeply threatened. In such a reactive state a person behaves automatically until they regain composure. Trances, as we discussed, are a profound loss of free will. Whatever you did in the trance may make you feel guilty later on, after you calm down.

Identifying when you slip into these automatic trance states, and learning how to prevent them helps you recover significantly more control over your life and outbursts. I spoke to one of my professors, Dr. Ugo Galgiardi, from Harvard about what had happened with the investors. He gave me this advice: "Never do anything when you are emotional." I took his advice. It took me awhile to calm down and realize everything was going to be okay again. Then I re-approached the situation with fresh eyes. Since then I've come to believe his advice as very useful in many walks of life. It's also true in eating. Ayurveda says never to eat when you are emotional, even if you are hungry. Eating while emotional causes indigestion, and overeating. Instead, always take the time to deal with your emotions first.

To help you wake up from a compulsive trance that makes you overeat, and to prevent them from reoccurring, it's useful to study the trance. Think of it as a separate personality, and then to identify the thoughts, feelings and emotions that are active in that state. You can ask this alternative personality questions. Is it an angry personality? A sad personality? An anxious personality? How would you describe this personality? What triggered your trance? How did you feel physically before you were triggered? Ayurveda believes that emotional states are related to your physical state. You might be feeling exhausted or tired. You might be simply hypoglycemic. When hypoglycemic, people tend to lose all control and have to go to the vending machine to get candy or snacks. You might be having digestive problems or be constipated. Digestive disorders make a person very anxious. Your heart may be strained by stress or congested blood. You might have a sinus infection. Any of these imbalances can make you more emotionally sensitive and trigger compulsive overeating.

Try to identify when your trance is triggered. Your body and mind have a natural rhythm to them. For some people, their compulsive overeating happens at the same time every day. Try to identify the time of day that you get the craving to binge. Normally, people tend to eat compulsively during an afternoon slump or at night time. You may feel abandonment or loneliness just before going to bed, and as a result may reach for food to comfort or soothe you.

People who eat compulsively overindulge in several ways. Some people have an addiction to a particular food that is bad for them, such as a sugar addiction. They feel compelled to eat that particular food often. Other people struggle with compulsive overeating in general, which means they have trouble limiting the quantity of food they eat. Some people binge eat. Binging is eating past the point when you are comfortably full, often in a rushed and emotional manner. It is related to compulsive eating. Binging is when you come home and start digging through the pantry, eating everything in sight until you are extremely full and cannot eat anymore. Binging includes eating excessive amounts of a single food, like eating a whole cheesecake by yourself or a whole bag of jumbo chips in one sitting. Often, during a binge, a person feels out of control and like they have no way of slowing down or stopping their behavior. People also often binge on processed or junk foods, but not always. Of the different types of addiction, binging triggers the most guilt and shame in general.

Finally there is grazing - when a person picks at food throughout the day. With grazing, you may never have a full belly. You may eat and eat and eat all day long and even though you've eaten enough calories for your body, you never get the satisfaction of good solid meal - so you just keep on eating. This perhaps seems like the mildest of food addictions, but thinking about and picking at food all day can be just as debilitating as any other food addiction. Working to eat three solid meals a day and cutting back on snacking can really be a big help.

People struggling through addictions often feel like they are weak-willed. If you are struggling with a food addiction, you might think, "I know I shouldn't have eaten that cookie, but I did. I have no willpower." But addiction generally isn't merely a lack of willpower or discipline. The root of the addiction is often a physical or psychological imbalance. You can't just fight the addiction; you also have to address the original cause of the addiction. Of course, willpower and discipline have an important role to play in your life. But when it comes to compulsive or addictive type of behaviors - you must address the root cause. Without addressing the cause, your willpower will be under constant attack from underlying psychological drives. Discipline is important, but it does not treat the real root causes. A healthy combination of self-inquiry and inner work along with discipline can eventually lead to a healing of these behaviors.

Denial

The trouble with false hungers is that people are generally in denial about them or defensive, even when they know they have a problem. They say, "I'm not really addicted to cigarettes, or food, or alcohol, or work...I can stop any time I want." But that's not the reality. The reality is that they can't stop.

If a person is in denial, they become defensive when anyone suggests abstinence from the food, the drug, the alcohol - whatever it is they are wanting. They may respond with, "What? Why are you nagging me? Or telling me I can't eat this food?!" Challenging their addiction brings outrage and indignation. "Let me be free. If you tell me to eat something, I'm just going to do the opposite." They try to justify their decision, by saying something like, "I deserve this," or "at least it doesn't have corn syrup." This kind of defensive response is natural when a person feels ashamed of themselves and their addictions. They become rebellious because they don't want to feel the shame. They don't want to admit that what they are doing is wrong and hurtful to themselves and others.

What are some ways that you defend yourself when you have eaten something you know you shouldn't? What are the excuses you give? Is there anyone that you blame for eating the way that you do? How do you convince yourself that this time is an exception to the rule?

I once had a client who said to me, "I don't have to fit the magazine image. I'm going to eat cake anyway because I'm beautiful no matter how much I weigh." There's nothing wrong with eating cake. And, believing that you are beautiful is healthy and important. But the reality was that this client didn't feel beautiful on the inside, and she felt guilty for eating the cake. She was trying to convince herself instead of acknowledge her inner feelings. It became clear that this client was struggling with their body image and eating the cake amounted to self-sabotage and self-loathing. It's hard to believe, but everyone engages in self-sabotage to some extent, often for mysterious reasons. If you are in denial about this self-sabotage, you will become a rebel. By rebelling you don't have to face the failure. If you justify the piece of cake then you don't have to really face the false hunger and the emotions behind it. Step 4 of Alcoholics Anonymous requires that you fearlessly search and make a moral inventory of your actions. By accepting responsibility of self-sabotage, you suddenly discover you can choose to treat yourself and others well again.

Of the three body types in Ayurveda, denial is Kapha is nature. Some kapha people do not like to feel their emotions, because they are over stimulating. Kapha people also tend to have water retention. When they feel emotions, it stimulates their circulatory system and movement of this water. A person with water retention cries easily, gets flushed when they have an emotion, and may feel breathless. All of this causes them to panic when they feel emotions, so they don't want to feel them. They prefer to remain in denial. If a person tends to get stuck in denial, getting rid of excess water weight can help make your emotions easier to face. Eat a low sodium diet. Include diuretics in your diet such as celery, parsley and asparagus. Once the excess water is flushed from their system, they will be able to confront powerful emotions without getting overwhelmed. Limit red meat consumption and fried food, as these will create liver congestion, which can make emotions difficult to face. If you have trouble facing emotions, you can also try exercising or other activities to improve your circulation. The general rule of thumb with denial is to take actions that are cleansing and also those that remove obstacles.

As everyone knows in Alcoholics Anonymous, no one can overcome addiction on their own. So when you fail, don't judge yourself. Remember that it is OK to fail, but it is important to recognize it and not defend it. To admit failure is a great act of courage and humility. In Alcoholics Anonymous, they say that it's important that when you fail or mess up, you have to admit it to yourself, admit it to God, and admit it to one other person. There's a lot of wisdom in that because we're all going to fail. If you can admit your mistakes and learn from them you are far more likely to succeed at your goals.

If you have been compulsively overeating for some time, you may have developed a greater tolerance for eating large quantities of food. Increased tolerance is one of the signs and symptoms of addiction. An alcoholic can tolerate more alcohol than a non-alcoholic because their bodies have adjusted and compensate for the alcohol. As your body builds tolerance, over time it expects you to continue eating more and more sweets. Your body comes to expect that most of its calories will come from sugary foods, and you will feel starved if you suddenly eliminate sweets from your diet. When you are used to eating sweets all the time, your thyroid and pancreas adapt to having excessively sweet blood. Your body modifies enzyme production to optimize digestion of your meals. The ability of your body to adapt to your diet and eating habits is a sign of your body's incredible biological intelligence. But once your body goes through this process it wants you to stick to the status quo. Once your body builds tolerance, the addiction is harder to overcome because it is no longer merely psychological, but it is also a physical addiction.

Did you ever notice you wake up ravenous after a large meal? Tolerance increases after a large meal. This effect is more noticeable after a heavy carbohydrate meal. A large meal makes you feel hungry the next morning because blood sugar levels spike after a large meal. When they drop again after the meal is digested, a person experiences symptoms of "relative hypoglycemia." One of these symptoms is increased appetite. The day after a large meal, you will feel as if your stomach is completely empty, and you may feel very hungry.

Studies also show that binge eating and repeated large meals increases stomach capacity, increasing tolerance.[12] One of my clients had a Russian grandma who forced her to eat beyond her capacity when she was a baby. Her grandma would always say, "Two milks," meaning she had to drink two bottles. Her grandma had

---

12 Allan Geliebter & Sami A. Hashim, "Gastric Capacity in normal, obese, and bulimic women," *Physiology & Behavior,* 74 (2001): 743 – 746.

experienced poverty and food insecurity herself as a child, and wanted her granddaughter to be hearty and plump. My client was habituated to overeating and felt uncomfortable when her stomach was empty. Even as an adult, she had trouble regulating portions. You might have grown up in a family where you were expected to eat everything on your plate, regardless of your hunger, fullness, and satiety cues. Then as an adult, you find yourself struggling to hear to your body's internal appetite cues, and eat beyond your capacity habitually. Perhaps you eat beyond your capacity because you eat too quickly or while distracted.

One of the biggest appetite regulators of your body is the feeling of a full stomach. The stomach is a muscular bag with many folds that stretches when you eat. After a normal meal the stomach expands to 1 liter (0.26 gallon), however during a large meal it can stretch up to 4 liters to accommodate an entire gallon of food. Normally, stuffing your stomach beyond the 1 liter capacity can make you feel tired and nauseous, causing pain & discomfort, and leading to heartburn. When a person eats excessive portions chronically, tolerance increases and they need to eat larger portions to feel satiated. Chronic overstuffing also reduces pain sensitivity when full.[13] Each time you eat too much and overstretch your stomach, your stomach seems harder to fill the next time. Your body gets used to having an abnormally high amount of food in its stomach and you won't feel satisfied with normal portions. This is because a person with a large stomach capacity digests their food more slowly. Overstuffing causes peristalsis, the rhythmic contractions that propel food through your

13 A Geliebter, et al., "Gastric capacity, gastric emptying, and test meal intake in normal and bulimic women," *American Journal of Clinical Nutrition* (1992), 56: 656–661.

GI, to slow or stop. When digestive function slows down and it reduces hormones like CCK (cholecystokinin) that make you feel satisfied.

Fortunately, eating normal portions can reverse this effect within four weeks, reducing gastric capacity by 27-36 percent, bringing tolerance levels back to normal.[14] Simply eat normal portions on a routine, and avoid snacking. This will help your blood sugar levels to stabilize, your pancreas and thyroid adjust to normal eating patterns, and your stomach capacity to self-regulate. Just like it took time for your body to develop tolerance to overeating give your body the time it needs to re-adjust to a new, healthy habit.

Once a person has developed a tolerance for overeating, they also experience withdrawal symptoms once they stop overeating. Withdrawal symptoms are one of the cardinal signs and symptoms of addiction. When a person is addicted to coffee, they get a headache if they don't drink it. When a person is addicted to food, they get anxious and irritable when they can't have food. If you suddenly stop snacking, you may feel hypoglycemic the first few weeks of abstinence. During the withdrawal phase, dopamine, the same neurotransmitter that makes you feel good when you eat sugar, declines. Then, your sense of well-being vanishes and you will experience the signs and symptoms of hypoglycemia: anxiety, irritability, confusion, shaky feeling, sweating, anger, and headaches. This is especially true for sugar withdrawal symptoms.

Just a few days ago, we took the kids out for ice-cream. The ice cream store offered regular ice cream and fat-free almond milk ice-cream. We started to wonder

14 A Geliebter, et al., "Reduced stomach capacity in obese subjects after dieting, "*American Journal of Clinical Nutrition* (1996); Feb 63 (2): 170-3.

whether it was better to eat the regular ice-cream or the fat-free version. Regular ice-cream is higher in calories, but is also more balanced nutritionally. It has more protein and fats. The almond milk was sugary like normal ice-cream, but not balanced by proteins and fats. We reasoned that the almond milk version would create a blood sugar spike because it did not have fat and protein to stabilize it. Instead of choosing the low calorie option, we chose the more balanced option. To offset the extra calories, we ordered a kiddie cone instead of an adult portion.

Low-fat foods were heavily advertised through the late 80s and 90s. However, many people on a low-fat diet compensate by eating more sweets and carbohydrates because they never feel satisfied. Refined carbs and simple sugars cause blood sugar and insulin to skyrocket. You will feel like you are on a blood sugar roller coaster as levels start to drop again, creating symptoms of hypoglycemia. We didn't want a sugar spike or the crash afterwards, so we avoided the low-fat option in the ice-cream store. In our home, we try to enjoy moderate portions of food with a balance of fats, proteins, & carbs, such as can be found naturally in whole foods. That way, we won't have to worry about withdrawal symptoms.

Many people know they have a food addiction, but have trouble abstaining because the symptoms of withdrawal are too intense. To boot, the feelings they were repressing with food all come to the surface. To minimize withdrawal symptoms, try reducing consumption slowly. Slow and steady always wins the race. It is important to not suddenly stop drinking coffee if you have been drinking 4-5 cups a day for years. It would be better to slowly reduce your consumption day by day so you don't shock your body. With sugar and snacking however, it may be better to cut it out cold turkey. However, you'll want to be sure that you are eating natural, healthy, and well-rounded meals so that your body feels safe and nourished, despite the big change. In short, don't cut out the "bad" stuff without adding in adequate "good" stuff.

Recognize that painful feelings and emotions are still likely to come up when you make a big change, and that is OK - healthy, in fact. We all want to avoid painful experiences. This survival instinct is healthy when it comes to injury. A natural response to pain, whether you've nicked your finger chopping vegetables or have been severely triggered emotionally, is to avoid repeating the painful experience. Similarly, you'll naturally want to avoid withdrawal symptoms because they can be painful. My herbal teacher, Frank Cook, used to say that feeling pain is feeling life. Only a dead person doesn't feel pain, or someone who has numbed themselves with food, alcohol, or drugs. But never make pain your enemy. If I cut myself with a knife, who is my enemy? The knife? Or the pain? The pain is not the enemy - it is your friend. It tells you what needs to be healed. Instead of avoiding your pain, try to see the pain and suffering of withdrawal as an opportunity; an opportunity to grow. Pain shows you what you need to heal. If you numb that experience, you miss your chance to grow. And normally, your withdrawal symptoms will only last 2-5 days. For some people it is longer and for others it is shorter, but it won't last forever. Like everything in this life, it will come and go.

Once you are ready to confront withdrawal symptoms, the following recommendations will help you heal from food addiction. Avoid processed and refined foods, especially foods containing sugar, corn syrup, and trans-fats. Avoid foods that come in a box if they have more than 5 ingredients in them, or some of the ingredients are chemicals instead of farm foods. Exercise caution with low-fat or fat-free foods. If you buy these foods, make sure they aren't substituting sugar for fats. Cut out coffee, and if possible, alcohol and smoking. Avoid snacks with refined sugar or carbohydrates. If you really feel like your body needs a snack, a handful of raw almonds or a piece of fruit will suffice.

To help you avoid temptation, clean out your cupboard of all processed foods. Then, stock your kitchen with natural, whole foods only. People often say that they feel like they need to buy processed foods for their husband, or wife, or children. If this is the case, have a conversation with your family about a dietary shift in the household. That's essential to your health and well-being. Explain they are welcome to eat those foods outside of the home. Select foods that are healthy for your unique body constitution. Eat a diet with plenty of fiber and greens. Choose nutritious meals that have balanced proportions of carbohydrates, fats, and proteins.

Bitter herbs like neem can help you reduce the effects of sugar withdrawal. An herbal tea brewed with ginger & cardamom can help you wean from coffee. Ginger and cardamom also wakes you up, helping you to feel bright and lively. Detoxification can dramatically reduce withdrawal symptoms. To help your body quickly detox from poor food choices, drink CCF tea (cumin coriander & fennel tea) throughout the day. This mild diuretic will flush toxins out through your kidneys. A ½ tsp of triphala in warm water at night is a mild laxative that will also help you flush out toxins.

One of the most powerful ways to help you overcome food addiction is with a *panchakarma* cleanse. A *panchakarma* cleanse is an Ayurvedic cleansing technique that is famous for its ability to deeply and safely cleanse your body. A *panchakarma* cleanse will not only help you overcome your addiction physically, but it will also help you overcome your addiction emotionally. A full *panchakarma* cleanse isn't something you can do at home, but you can do a modified version. To enjoy the benefits of a *panchakarma* cleanse, find a professional Ayurvedic practitioner or spa to guide you.

Take time to plan your meals at the beginning of each day, so you don't slip back into addictive habits. If possible, cook all your meals before leaving for work in the morning. You can refrigerate meals for later or keep them warm in a crock pot until dinner. Get enough sleep, exercise, and water. Eat only when you are truly hungry. Eat slowly and mindfully so that you can regulate portions without effort. Learn how to cope with stress without using food to self-soothe. These are simple and healthy food habits that we all know are good for us.

Conclusion

*   *   *

We are each born with an understanding of how to feed and take care of ourselves, but unfortunately this knowing gets lost along the way. We lose touch with our inner knowing; we question our cravings and appetite, and start looking externally for answers. We go on diets, cut out carbs or fats or proteins, or get a lap band surgery or liposuction. But none of these strategies get you back to the root of the problem, or back in touch with your hunger. This book is an attempt to guide you back to that pure wisdom and self-knowledge, hidden in your hunger, that leads to true health and well-being.

There is no formula for weight loss, how to be healthy, or how to find peace with food. No one, no expert, and certainly no diet has the secret to weight loss. Weight loss is a personal and inner journey, not a formula. The best and brightest dietitian or Ayurvedic practitioner can give you some ideas and basic guidelines, but ultimately the truth and knowledge of how to eat for your unique body type lies only within you. This shouldn't disappoint you. Rather, this news is uplifting. Like any spiritual awakening, discovering how to be healthy is part of your unique life story, and your personal inner journey. This journey is an exciting one.

We are all pilgrims through life, and one of the most joyous activities of life is personal growth. You get to write your own novel and solve your own mystery.

In this book, you have explored all the nuances of hunger. You have learned about appetite, food cravings, emotional hunger, desire, and food addiction. You have learned about hunger from a biological, emotional, and spiritual angle. It is our hope that through your awareness of hunger from a cognitive approach, you will be more aware of your relationship to food, and better able to make healthy choices for YOUR specific body. We have helped you move beyond knowledge of diets, food, and calories to an inner experience of your hunger. Use this experience to guide you. It is also our hope that by exploring and experiencing your hunger, emotions and desires, you will come to develop the strength to delay gratification.

All that we have been talking about - all the knowledge and wisdom you have learned about food and your body - will be for naught unless you can apply your new knowledge and experience into real behavior change. What is the special formula that can help you make this transition? There are two essential ingredients that will give you the power to transform your life.

The first of these is vigilance. What is the nature of this vigilance and how should one apply it? This is the vigilance to stay awake, to remain aware and to self-examine. It is tempting to fall asleep and gloss over the consequences of your actions and the details of your life. But then you will miss your life! Apply your vigilance to recognizing the ways in which your relationship with food is keeping you from achieving your full potential in life.

The second of these is the discipline to hope. Hope isn't something that comes naturally. You have to do it. Hope, like love, isn't a feeling but a verb. When you have hope, you also have motivation to succeed. You must practice hoping for it to become alive within you. You must cultivate the skills to hope, even in hopeless situations. Where you have hope, you have passion and willpower, and then magic happens. Hopelessness is the greatest evil to health. It is the source of all emptiness and false hungers, and you must use vigilance to fight hopelessness in all its forms. Armed with the vigilance to discover yourself, and the discipline to hope, you will transform your entire life, and achieve a healing from within.

Imagine if you could take all of the energy you spend thinking about food, diet, and your body and direct it towards something meaningful that you believe in. This could be your family, friends, loved ones, your occupation, an important cause. The world and the people around you need you to be you! Replace those thoughts about food and your body with something positive. This is why all of us are called to heal - so that we can truly give and devote ourselves fully to one another and be more present for our lives.

So, we will leave this question to you: How will you satisfy your hunger? Now that you know hunger, what will you eat?

65369069R00101

Made in the USA
Lexington, KY
10 July 2017